Memoirs of a
Cotswold
Vet

Memoirs of a Cotswold Vet

Ivor Smith BVSc MRCVS

For Angela

First published 2008

The History Press Ltd
The Mill, Brimscombe Port
Stroud, Gloucestershire, GL5 2QG
www.thehistorypress.co.uk

British Library Cataloguing in Publication Data.
A catalogue record for this book is available from the British Library.

ISBN 978 0 7509 5108 1

Typesetting and origination by The History Press Ltd.
Printed in Great Britain

CONTENTS

ACKNOWLEDGEMENTS

Not having written a book before, I find it difficult to know where to begin acknowledging the large number of wonderful people who have been part of my life and most of my story, for without them there would be no story. First and foremost thanks must go to the animals, most of whom were cooperative patients. Some, however, were outrageously uncooperative, and these were often the ones that made the most memorable stories. For better or for worse, most of the animals had owners, and without them some of the chapters in this book would be less lively.

I was lucky enough to have had generous parents and an exceptional aunt who encouraged learning. Unfortunately, as a youngster I succumbed to a serious illness that resulted in my absence from school for almost a year. Ironically, in view of my later profession, the doctors believed that the infection had been passed to me via one of my menagerie of pets and ordered all of them to be destroyed, with the sole exception of my dog, Nellie. It was probably at this defining moment that I decided I wanted to know all there was to know about diseases of animals and how to put them right. I cannot remember a time when I did not want to be a vet.

My family ensured that I would continue to be taught at home and no doubt this was an enormous help when I returned to my primary school, and eventually resulted in me progressing to grammar school.

Life at the Crypt School in Gloucester was hard work and discipline was strict. I believe that most of the masters were truly dedicated and I appreciated what I achieved through them. There are two staff members I feel compelled to name. There have been occasions when I have been reminded that the purpose of my Crypt School education was not how to be taught to play rugby, this ridiculous game where at a very early age you walk from the field with a bloody nose and decades later your assailant is still a close friend. Our outstanding master of sport who put us through this agony was Horace Edwards. He taught me, and hundreds of other lads, that there is far more to life than scoring tries.

Charles Lepper was our English master who, for many years, excelled in producing our school's nationally famed Shakespearean dramas. If acting was not your forte his endless energy taught hundreds of lesser mortals like me how to enjoy literature and, possibly, how to write a book!

The teaching staff at Liverpool University's Faculty of Veterinary Science were mainly excellent, and some truly brilliant. We were of course at that age when we criticised everything and knew just how to resolve every problem in the world. In professional life I had only two bosses and I benefited from the company and professionalism of my Cheltenham principal, Peter Hull.

In my thirty years as principal of The Brambles Veterinary Practice in Churchdown, it has been a privilege and pleasure to have enjoyed the company of so many dedicated people, including Sue, Angie and Claire among others, whose efforts over three decades I truly appreciated.

Last, but by no means least, I must mention a dedicated member of staff without whom this story would be incomplete. I was indeed fortunate at an early time in my life to meet my wife Angela, someone who shared the same interests as me and without whom these *Memoirs of a Cotswold Vet* would have been very different.

INTRODUCTION

Writing a book relating to my veterinary career was something I had never considered until I was approached by Matilda Richards, a commissioning editor at a local publishing company, at the end of a talk I had given that mainly revolved around the village of Churchdown – where I had 'put up my plate' in 1972.

While preparing for the talk I reflected on some of the events that led me to contemplate starting my own practice. I began to realise just how much had happened during my life and how much of it was a mix of success and failure. The more I thought about the past, the more recollections vividly returned to mind.

I realised with amazement that in one ten-year period I had gone from being an eleven-year-old at junior school to a twenty-one-year-old on the brink of getting married. Not every decade was quite as eventful as that, but a life spent with animals made sure that there were few dull days.

My life began in Birmingham at the height of the Second World War blitz and many hours of my earliest years were spent in the safety and indignity of an air-raid shelter. My family moved to Gloucester in 1945 and I became a pupil at Finlay Road School – at that time one of Gloucester's best-performing schools. From there that I moved on to the Crypt School in the city, and eventually to the Faculty of Veterinary Science at Liverpool University. There I gained my Bachelor of Veterinary Science degree and became a veterinary surgeon.

I have written here a little about undergraduate life at the university. It was a time when students were genuinely hard-up and under the continual stress of learning and taking exams that had to be passed. Fortunately you were not on your own and the pressures were shared in the company of a small group of students who were experiencing the same stress. It was amazing how a pint, a chat and a laugh in our local pub kept our spirits up.

I was particularly fortunate in having a special mate to cheer me up. In the middle of what seemed a never-ending course, Angela, my longstanding Gloucestershire girlfriend, and I married at St Philip and St James's Church, Hucclecote, in 1963.

Not surprisingly most of my vet student year grew to become lifelong friends. I have written a little about a few of them but it would have been easy to have related something of interest of them all. At least I have spared their blushes.

I began my first job at a veterinary practice in Crudwell, Wiltshire, in 1966 – it was a fast learning curve being a young veterinary surgeon. My boss was unique and I have tried to describe what life with him was like. Although it is fair to say he would never get away with it today, he did provide some incredible memories. When I left his practice, I joked to friends at the time that if I ever wrote a book, half of it would be devoted to my first two years in the Crudwell practice. I have, however, resisted that temptation and restricted the telling of those days in order to include equally fascinating happenings at different times and in different places.

From Crudwell we moved to Cheltenham. It was towards the end of the Swinging Sixties and there was just a short while to let our hair down before life became much more serious and demanding. For many years I had a superb boss. Peter Hull is greatly respected in the veterinary profession, his farming clients and the pet owners, and extensively throughout the horse world. I enjoyed his company and, from our good-humoured chats that sometimes resembled a lecture over a cup of coffee, I continued to learn a great deal about the art and science of veterinary practice. We parted company when I left his practice and, with his blessing, moved to Churchdown to start my own practice. However, he has remained a good friend to this day.

We had bought The Brambles, a large, cold Victorian house into which Angela and I, our toddler son and our dog moved in January 1972. By the end of that first rewarding year, we had a daughter too, a surgery and a house with central heating. The practice continued to grow and the following thirty years whizzed by, but not without leaving behind many memorable tales.

By the time I retired in 2001 it had become necessary to build new premises to accommodate the ever-increasing numbers of staff. It was also an opportunity to provide state-of-the-art facilities for the growing numbers of clients and their pets. So, in August 1999, The Brambles Veterinary Practice moved across the road to its new hospital-type home. Many dedicated people have worked for the practice over the years and life would not have been the same without their company. I have written about some and, if it was possible, I would have mentioned the contribution of many more, but they are all an essential part of my story. It has been a challenge to decide which of the often astonishing events in my life to include and which to leave out.

Invariably while sitting around a dining table, the stories of the animals and day-to-day practice life have been related to friends who have always seemed eager to hear them. I am frequently surprised when they remind me of amusing events that happened years before, and I sometimes have difficulty recalling them myself. Some, of course, are remembered because they were especially sad.

In places I have changed the names of certain people in order to protect their identity. It is not my intention to portray anyone in a misleading light and I apologise to those who may feel this is the case.

I have tried to find a balance between the contrasting types of stories and I hope that I have succeeded. The leading players have, naturally, been my patients, and without them I would not have a story to tell.

Ivor Smith, 2008

CHAPTER ONE

ONCE UPON A TIME IN A COTSWOLD VILLAGE

The telephone rang in the old farmhouse. My wife, Angela, picked it up and a few moments later called to me in the garden.

'Ive, can you have a word with Mr Pitt from Poole Keynes? He thinks he might need you to calve a cow.'

'Okay. With you in a minute Ange', I yelled back, and left my spade upright in the soggy soil. I was thinking that it never seemed to stop raining around here.

This was the call I had been dreading. It was September 1966. I had been a qualified veterinary surgeon for eight weeks and the principal of the practice had decided that I could probably be trusted to run the place for a few hours on my own. Just in case there was a total catastrophe, he had given me several numbers where I might be able to get in touch with him. One was the local rugby club. One was a pub. One was a hotel/pub. I was uncertain about the fourth.

I picked up the phone and said hello to Mr Pitt and sorry we hadn't met before. He apologised for bothering me on a Saturday afternoon. The compliments exchanged, Farmer Pitt explained that the cow in question was due to calve: she had been straining for a couple of hours but was making no progress.

'I've had a feel inside', he volunteered, as farmers do on these occasions, 'and I can only feel an 'ead.'

'Lord, I hope I can feel a bit more than that', I thought to myself. 'I'll be with you as soon as I can Mr Pitt', I told the farmer. 'I'll be about twenty minutes.'

Everything I could possibly need on this assignment was checked three times. I hoped my client would provide the soap and towel. Off I roared in the practice's muddy blue Ford Cortina. Less than twenty minutes later I stood nobly in my rubber calving gown behind my patient; my arms and the rear end of the cow were swathed in soap. Now was the moment of bubbly truth. My hand explored the unknown.

Like Farmer Pitt I too could feel a head, and what's more I could also feel a foot, well, one foot anyway. With a bit more soap and a lot of slippery lubricant my hand slid around the calf and down to the missing backward-pointing leg. A slim clean rope was passed round the calf's fetlock, and gentle traction, with my hand cupping the foot to protect the wall of the uterus, brought the limb to its proper position. After that it was plain sailing. With a rope round the other leg and a few hefty pulls, the calf slid into our world.

As I scrubbed up in cold water, I glowed inside with satisfaction watching the little heifer calf suckling from her mum. Not bad for a first attempt. I believe the sentiments applied to both of us.

'No, I won't stop for a drink Mr Pitt, but thanks anyway.'

Back in the car, with headlights and swishing windscreen wipers on, and heading for our Crudwell farmhouse home, my thoughts travelled back to the events of the last decade. So much had happened. I pondered upon the ups and downs that we had already experienced. 'Well, the last ten years have been damned hard going but I think I'm going to enjoy this job', I said out loud. I'm sure I'm not the only person in the world who talks to himself.

Forty years on and I have rarely regretted that momentous decision to become a vet. In truth I don't think there was ever a *single* momentous occasion. As a Gloucester youngster I grew up with animals of all shapes and sizes, courtesy of very tolerant parents, and I think that the idea of spending my life working with them probably grew with me. At one stage our home was shared by the obligatory dog and cat of course, but also in attendance were the pet mice, hamsters, guinea pigs, a rabbit, tropical fish, cold water fish, pond fish, frogs, newts and slow-worms. I bet I've missed somebody out.

Disaster struck in late 1947. Many people still associate that year with a dreadful winter and snowdrifts that appeared mountainous to youngsters. The spectacular floods that followed the melting of the snow added to the miseries of many local folk, but, in true British fashion and more than a bit of Gloucester humour, the adversities, as usual, were overcome.

My problems were a bit different. A few weeks before Christmas I developed an illness that almost put an end to me. My medical records state I had polio-meningitis, and at one stage it was touch and go, so they say. Nobody knew how I became infected, but just in case it originated from one of our menagerie of animals, the doctors instructed my father to have all my pets put to sleep. Only my dog was spared. She was Nellie.

I have no idea why anyone would want to call their dog Nellie but when dad brought her home she came with a name, and for many happy years old Nel was a prominent member of our family. Most of the time I thought this black and white sort of Border Collie cross was the most popular member of the family. Seeing her face on the wintry side of the hospital ward window on Christmas Day certainly cheered me up. Perhaps soon they might let me go home, and I couldn't wait to get better and be with her. Walks with Nel on Robinswood Hill would never be the same again. There was no doubt in my mind she would be my best mate forever, and she was – until my thirteenth birthday anyway.

Had the events of that year initiated the vet vocation journey? Who knows? I can only say that if I close my eyes I can recall countless details of that very strange time in my life.

I was a pupil at Gloucester's Finlay Road School, recognised then as one of the city's leading junior schools. The majority of the children in the school passed 'the Scholarship' exam, later to become known as the 11 plus, and left to go to the grammar school, or any other school of their choice. At this time a strange anomaly was the relative ease of winning a place at a Gloucester grammar school if you lived within the city boundary. It had one of the highest intakes in the country. If you lived outside the boundary the opposite was the case, and it was difficult to get into a grammar school. The unsuccessful pupils went to one of the city's secondary modern schools. There was just one thing wrong with these schools – their description. They were modern but the term 'secondary' erroneously and daftly suggested the pupils were second-class students, to some people anyway. Consequently, there was a high proportion of very bright articulate youngsters at most of the schools.

Life at Finlay Road was an enjoyable time with a wonderful teaching staff that were particularly helpful to me following a nine-month absence recovering from polio-meningitis (if such it was). Sadly, fifty years on, life has not been kind to the school; it has recently been described as an 'underperformer' and, at the time of writing, is 'up for sale' by Gloucestershire County Council. No doubt there is still plenty of the old Gloucester spirit to turn things round.

I left my junior school in 1952 with many happy memories and friends and moved on to the Crypt, Gloucester's oldest grammar school. Founded in 1539, the Crypt was, of course, a lot younger when I attended. Getting to school was fun; we rode our bikes. In fact we seemed to ride our bikes everywhere back then. For many of us this was after we had finished our paper round. Delivering early morning papers was the acknowledged way of having a schoolboy income. The 5s wage did not go far but at least made it possible to invite a girl to the pictures, just in case she didn't offer to pay for herself. Most mornings I was awake enough to glance at the papers' headlines as I pushed them through the letterboxes. One day was paramount; it was indeed the day the music died. That was 3 February 1959. Buddy Holly had been killed in an airplane crash.

There seemed no urgent need for girlfriends in 1952 although we boys talked about them a great deal. Getting to know your new schoolmates seemed sufficiently rewarding for the time being, without knowing of course that some of these boys would become your lifelong friends. Learning French, Latin and Greek all at the same time was daunting but we seemed to cope. Maths, English, history, geography and the sciences were thrown in for good measure. Somehow there was still time to fit in the weekly periods of religious instruction, music and a session in the gym, plus the all-important weekly afternoon of sport.

In our first school year every subject was compulsory, and that included our introduction to the game of rugby football. Our Welsh rugby-international games master, Horace Edwards, must have despaired at his attempts to teach us the new discipline. Most of us had come from junior schools where we had played football with a round ball and were reluctant to change codes. Nevertheless most had been converted within a few weeks. Our school tried its best to make gentlemen of us off the playing field, but permitted us to be hooligans when on it. At the start our skill levels allowed us to do little more than get plastered in mud. Everyone yelling as they got under the tepid shower after a game was a new experience.

The years passed quickly, and no sooner had we taken O-levels than the A-level exams upon which so much depended had arrived. The veterinary schools were happy with my grades and soon it was time to leave. Looking back on my school career, I could not complain about the teaching staff. For me they had done their job. Discipline was rigid, but most of us had benefited as a result, although today some of the methods employed by masters to enforce it would definitely be frowned upon.

For instance, Mr Morris, the woodwork master (who also taught maths) had his own way of ensuring your full concentration in class. Default and he would take you on a 'bicycle ride'. This entailed him grasping your 'sideboards' and twiddling the hair between his fingers in opposite directions. It was uncomfortable but it worked. We quickly learnt to listen and concentrate.

Our French master, Mr Fred Askew, employed his own methods too. At some stage during each lesson at least one boy would be asked, 'Aimez-vous Marie-Anne?' You quickly latched on that Marie-Anne was the big walloping stick our teacher carried. Get the question wrong and your hand was introduced to her personally. Today Mr Askew's teaching methods would be ridiculed and no doubt we would be hearing about impending legal action. Mr Askew, like so many teachers at that time, was, I suppose, an eccentric, but to suggest he was sadistic would be laughable. He was there to teach, and every lad who was fortunate enough to be in his class certainly learnt some French. Fifty years on and I have yet to meet any of his pupils who do not look back if not with approval, then at least with a degree of fondness.

Our Crypt School education was second to none. Every boy had achieved something. We joke today that our school had given us the social skills necessary for us to be welcomed anywhere in the world – at least on the first occasion. *Vivat Scholar Cryptiensis!*

My fondest memories of school will always be those of athletics and rugby. I was blessed with the ability to run fast and I left the Crypt possessing the records for both the 100- and 220-yard sprints. This had little to do with training me to become a vet, but friends have frequently wisecracked that this skill must have allowed me to get to the field gate before the bull. On more than one occasion they would be right, and if it wasn't the bull chasing me, it was something else (but, with hand on heart, I don't think it was ever the animal's owner!).

Rugby may have started from reluctant beginnings but it quickly developed into a passion that has remained a part of my life – perhaps I should say *our lives*, because for better or for worse my wife has always been part of this rugby world.

From the beginning of 1957, most Friday nights found me with a group of my classmates at the local youth club. These were the exciting days of Bill Haley, Elvis Presley and Buddy Holly. It hadn't taken me long to spot a very attractive fourteen-year-old young lady with a fashionable long ponytail, and the teenage crush followed. Her name was Angela. There was a bonus attraction. I knew via a good school pal who happened to be going out with her elder sister that their family owned one of the biggest televisions in the village. So on a cold Friday night in February, after a couple of hours of rocking and bopping, and knowing that England were taking on France at Twickenham the following afternoon, I chatted my way into joining them in their lounge the next day to watch the game on their big black and white box. I reckon you could say it was a successful first date – England won 9 points to 3. We could never have guessed on that occasion that we would still be watching rugby games on television together fifty years later.

During my final year at school I went for interviews at three veterinary schools in England. My third interview was at the University of Liverpool's Faculty of Veterinary Science. At the head of the table was seated the Dean, John George Wright, an eminent professor of veterinary medicine and surgery. I was asked to sit, and faced him at the other end. Between us sat six professors and other veterinary academic icons. JG, as he was affectionately known throughout the profession, welcomed me, made several humorous comments relating to what he already knew about me, and immediately put me at ease. The next half-hour flashed by and I hoped I had said enough to impress. I had, it seemed, and after a few moments conferring with the academics, the head of the table offered me a place. In 1960 the places, as now, were like gold dust, and to this day I cannot believe what came next.

'Thank you, sir', I replied, 'but I'd like to think about it.'

It was a moment of madness and must have made me seem remarkably cocky. It wasn't meant to sound as though I was playing hard to get, and I am sure I was simply thinking of the provisional place that one of the other schools had offered me. It took the entire group by surprise, myself included, and for a moment I wondered who would be the first to fall off his chair. It was my first real lesson that there are some things in life you just never say, and it could have meant the end of my veterinary career before it had even started. Perhaps the dignitaries were amused by my *faux pas* for, as promised, the treasured offer arrived in the post two days later. I only needed two minutes to consider the offer while I looked for my pen, then signed the acceptance form and ran to the nearest postbox.

My university career began later that year, but first there was a long summer holiday to get through. It was not a holiday in the usual sense. The urgency was to get a job. Any old job would do. The next five years would be hard going on a meagre income. But help was at hand via a friend. The friend in this case was one Keith Russell, a school pal I had grown up with. His dad, Wally, was an ex-Army serviceman who continued the war fighting in the scrum for Gloucester's Coney Hill Rugby Club. From Monday to Friday he was the general foreman of a well-known local building company. From time to time building things didn't go to plan and in fact some things went disastrously wrong, but Wally was always there to sort the problems out. Why they arose in the first place he never explained but that's another story, and it was all part of my education.

For the next three months I became a Gloucester navvy, digging, shovelling, mixing and wheelbarrowing. My partners in crime were literally that. They were three local lads who had served time for burglary and freely admitted it. One morning, while we sat on old boxes and bags of cement enjoying our ten-minute tea break, one of my new mates pulled out some crumpled old cuttings from his wallet. They had been taken from the Gloucester *Citizen* and were reports with pictures of various 'jobs' that they could personally relate to. My initial reaction was one of disbelief but the situation became almost comical as they started to criticise the paper's crime reporter for getting his facts wrong! Ironically, we were working at the time in Gloucester's historic Westgate

Street, refurbishing and rebuilding the Court Houses and Rooms. Naively, I thought it strange that they were on such familiar terms with the local uniformed police, and they were happy to introduce me to the plain–clothed detectives to whom they chatted informally. It took me a while to realise that they were established customers of the force.

Work on the building site was physically demanding, and we had targets to meet. We were a team and in some way the challenge had a bonding effect. It is interesting to note that, twenty–five years later, one of our gang was to become a regular sheep–farming client of my practice, for whom I have high regard.

October soon arrived and at last I was in Liverpool ready to begin the veterinary adventure. It took just a short while to adjust to the big city and northern life. I quickly made new friends and the Faculty of Veterinary Science just as quickly made it clear that the course we had embarked on was going to be increasingly demanding. We attended formal lectures five–and–a–half days a week interspersed with practical work. The twenty-nine lads and six female students in our year were split into groups of three for the practical sessions. For most of the time I was in the company of Roger Salmon and Nigel Sladen. We are still close friends today, having survived what seemed an eternal veterinary course together. Until their recent retirement, both Roger and Nigel spent their veterinary careers in Lancashire practices, though not the same one. Perhaps they should have, for during our years of studying veterinary anatomy, one had dissected the left side of a horse, the other the right. We concluded that eventually, to be fair to the client, they should go into practice together, so that when asked to visit an ailing horse, the practice receptionist could ask, 'Which side of the horse seems to be the problem?'

There was of course some time for us to do the things that students have always done. We put the world to rights in the Students' Union bar, ate egg and chips for lunch there most days, and lunched at one of Liverpool's 250 Chinese restaurants on a Friday. At our favourite venue a three-course meal with coffee was on offer for just 2s 1d. You could select very different-sounding dishes from the menu which, strangely, all tasted much the same, but was filling nonetheless.

The students organised the faculty Saturday night dance by rota. The disco had not yet been invented in the early 1960s and the live band was the order of the day. There was no shortage of them. How such a huge array of talented groups arose in the Liverpool area at that time will remain a mystery. The going rate to hire a band was around £20 and you could take your pick from Gerry and the Pacemakers to The Hollies; and yes, if you wanted them, The Beatles too.

Naturally I managed to fit in more than the odd game of rugby between my studies. The jump from the schoolboy game to the senior one was another culture shock. The gallantry seemed to have been left on the school playing fields and I soon realised getting tackled without the ball was part and parcel of this new version of the game. The excitement of university rugby was immense. The fixture list was impressive and included local club Sale! But this was the day of the amateur player and although a handful of Liverpool students had played for what are now Premiership sides, these teams at the time were rather different from the professional international outfits that entertain us today.

Nevertheless, it was an opportunity to play with some of the outstanding players of the day. One remarkable player was our outside half, Tom Brophy. Tom wasn't a big fellow but he was fast and everyone agreed 'he can turn on a sixpence'. The art of playing with him was to try and figure out in which direction he was going to go. He did not score a lot of tries himself, but he was a three-quarter's delight. When the defence was completely mesmerised and out of position he would simply part with the ball and let one of the other backs cross the line. I last saw Tom on a black and white television taking part in an international game in the 1960s. He was playing for England.

I made time for courting during my first year at university. At one point I had not seen Angela, my now long-term girlfriend, for six weeks when she agreed to come up to Liverpool for the weekend. The intention was that she would be entertained by me during the day in Derby Hall, the male students' residence, and at night sneaked into nearby Dale Hall, the ladies' hall of residence, courtesy of a couple of our year's daring female vet students.

I met Angela on the Saturday morning as she stepped on to the platform of Lime Street Station from the Gloucester express train. Ever understanding, she agreed that I should play for my rugby XV that afternoon. I played, and my game lasted just twenty minutes. I was knocked unconscious, suffered a cracked jaw, and spent the rest of our romantic weekend in Sefton General Hospital.

If you cannot stand or understand rugby and believe it is a game that could well be played without a ball – and there I agree you may have a point – I promise not to mention it again (not on a personal level anyway). After my university days were over I was no longer able to play the game seriously, as most of my weekends were taken up in the company of our four-legged friends. Getting shoved around by hefty cattle in a confined space was, I suppose you could say, just an extended part of the game, but from now on it would be without the intervention of a referee.

I remained as courtly as I could for three years, which necessitated frequent short weekend visits to Gloucester to visit Angela. The train fare was ridiculously expensive and I only did it the once. The second choice, a comfortable economical bus ride for 7s 6d, complete with an on-board coffee service and toilet facilities, seemed to accomplish a tour of England before finally reaching Gloucester. It was just too slow. By the time I reached my destination I felt it must be time to head back to Liverpool. There had to be a better way, and there was – I decided to thumb a lift. This was many students' preferred method of travel at the time and I rapidly developed hitch-hiking into a fine art. To be honest I enjoyed the challenge and the heady leap into the unknown.

In the 1960s, for all practical purposes, Liverpool seemed a lot further away than it is today. A good run in your car from Gloucestershire would take a minimum of five hours. Heading north from Gloucester the familiar route rolled off the tongue like poetry. You took the A38 towards Tewkesbury, then on to Worcester, Kidderminster, Bridgnorth, Wellington, Whitchurch and on to the Chester bypass. At this point the sights, sounds and even the smells were changing rapidly. The strong scent of Lever Brothers' soap and detergent factories at Port Sunlight signalled that you had reached Ellesmere Port, quaint Rock Ferry and mighty Birkenhead. Through the Mersey Tunnel tollgates, sudden darkness and hey presto: you were in Liverpool. It would be many weeks before I could once again enjoy the clean air and rural smells of farms, fresh hay and cattle in Gloucestershire.

It was more than good fortune that one of my year hailed from the Cainscross area of Stroud. Graham Hall had been educated at Stroud's Marling School, which just happened to be my school's arch-rival, but despite that we quickly became good pals. He also owned a car that he had inherited from his grandfather, who had purchased it in 1939; a sturdy and very reliable Morris 10. For the first three years of our course the terms began and ended with his car pulling up at the front door of my parents' Longlevens home. There was just the faintest odour of motor fuel and oil, which was more than outweighed by the welcoming scent of real leather seats.

Graham had been blessed with at least two exceptional qualities. One was the Wisdom of Solomon and the other the Patience of Job. Today I look back with embarrassment as I recall his arriving with a tidy car, empty except for his briefcase and a few books. He must have cringed as all available vacant space was taken up by my briefcase, text books, rugby kit, Dansette radio-record player combined, stack of vinyl records, guitar and a 120lb set of Spur barbel weight-training gear, not to mention my full-size horse skeleton. Fortunately the hefty clutter had little effect on the sturdy Morris.

A few miles out of Gloucester we passed the church tower at Norton. It seemed to be a point of special reference, for, once past it, our mutual sadness at leaving family and friends behind began to ebb. We started to chat and joke and began to anticipate the enjoyment of meeting our vet pals congregating once more in Liverpool. Every year we remarked on the changes to the scenery that had taken place in the space of a few weeks; the bare trees we had passed in March now greeted us with new green shoots and leaves of spring as we journeyed north a month later. The journey south was, of course, always more special. We were returning home; the end of the Christmas term was extra-special. The sight of Norton Church emerging from the dusk on a late December afternoon, with snow beginning to fall, was intoxicating.

I made the homeward journey from Liverpool to Gloucester on several occasions during the ten-week term. The hitch-hiking resulted in many adventures and at the same time offered the opportunity to meet some interesting people. One that springs to mind was a lorry driver who drove in all weather with his cabin windows wound down. One of the unwritten rules of getting a lift was to provide companionship to the driver on your journey together. It was considered the height of bad manners to nod off, but that would have been impossible with this particular chap. The cold draughts from the open windows whizzed past my ears and the driver apologised for my discomfort. He explained that he had been a rear gunner on a Lancaster bomber on air raids over Germany and his experiences had left him severely claustrophobic. I shivered, not from the cold, but from the thought of being cocooned in that Perspex shell for so many long hours, picked out and blinded by enemy searchlights and shot at from below with no means of escape.

It was indeed an opportunity to meet folk from all walks of life, and mostly I enjoyed the journeys. One thing I had in common with the majority of strangers who stopped to pick me up was a love of food. Some lorry drivers may well enjoy their legendary Yorkie bar, but one thing is certain, they all loved their traditional roadside breakfast. The transport café hardly needed signposting. I am certain the welcoming odour of bacon cooking on a hot grill wafted for miles, and it was hard not to drool as the lorry rolled on to the lorry park. Ten minutes later I would be at a table with the driver eating rashers of hot greasy bacon protruding from thick rounds of buttered white bread. Ketchup or HP Sauce was optional, but a mug of strong hot tea was definitely part of the early morning feast. Perhaps it was from years of practice, but the drivers seemed to have stomachs of iron as they tipped the almost scalding brew down their necks before lighting up their Woodbine. Then it was back on the road.

Time goes quickly when you are busy and the first three years of the course were over surprisingly fast. For the first two years I had lived in Derby Hall, and the third in a house off the famous Penny Lane, which I shared with my fellow navy-blue-donkey-jacket-clad students, Nigel and Roger. We continued to enjoy our extra-curricular activities, but found ourselves with increasingly less time in which to do it. Most nights were spent studying veterinary anatomy, biochemistry and physiology. At about 9 o'clock each night we would take a break together and have a cup of coffee and Marmite on toast. We talked about anything other than anatomy. Except on one memorable occasion, when we did.

We happened to be concentrating on the chicken, having already spent some of the best days of our lives learning the anatomical differences of every creature on board Noah's Ark. Well, at the very least the horse, cow, sheep, pig, goat, dog and the cat. Roger was already boiling the kettle when we joined him in the kitchen. He was about to make one of the most momentous pronouncements of his life.

'Do you know chaps', he proclaimed, with an authority that only he could muster, 'the chicken does not have an interparietal bone in its skull?'

We doubted whether any veterinary surgeon in the country knew of this earth-shaking fact. We split our sides laughing, wondering how, armed with this knowledge, we would change the world of poultry medicine. It was an opportunity to relieve the strain of studying the apparent absurdity of the details we were being asked to learn by having an hysterical five minutes. There were scores of these daft but important tension-relieving moments during our last year living together.

The third year of the course quickly came and went. Angela and I had planned to get married at this time, and we duly were, at St Philip and St James's Church, Hucclecote, in 1963. Angela moved up to Liverpool – the hitch-hiking had been fun but time-consuming, and it was time that could be put to more valuable use. Perhaps today we would simply have moved in together, but at that time to do so would have been considered outrageously socially unacceptable. There were also benefits in the veterinary world of being a 'married man'.

Our final year was spent out of Liverpool at a rural field station on the beautiful Cheshire Wirral peninsula. Here the Vet School staff did their best to lick us into shape before letting us loose on an unsuspecting public. There was no let-up in the number of daily lectures and there seemed no end to the quantity of medical facts you were expected to remember. Theory was interspersed with demonstrations and practical work in the cobbled yards, paddocks and classrooms of the old country house that we fondly knew as Leahurst. Now it was hands-on time, though no doubt a few of the animals probably wished we'd kept our hands to ourselves. The classic image of the farm vet is one of spending his day standing at the rear of a cow with one arm somewhere inside her. For those who have never dared ask why we actually do this, it is the basic examination for pregnancy. A competent vet will carry out this procedure quickly with the minimum of discomfort to the patient, but even the most experienced has to start somewhere, and it may well have been in a paddock at Leahurst.

This usually quick procedure, when first attempted, tends to be a more protracted affair and the student's first impression on inserting his or her arm is to encounter only a handful of slurry-like substance. Eventually the hand detects an enlargement of the cow's uterus, indicating pregnancy, and the student cries 'Eureka!' before it's the turn of the next in line. Needless to say, by the time the last of the six students in the group has attempted to detect signs of pregnancy, the poor cow is wishing we would all go home and give her some rest.

At the end of a taxing week, an amusing hour on Friday afternoon was often spent around a horse presented to us with no health history. For the purpose of the exercise students were not told if the animal was at Leahurst for an in-depth investigation for a serious complaint or just happened to be a healthy horse borrowed from a local riding school. It was amazing how our enquiring minds ran riot and by the end of the session we had suggested the early stages of just about every known disease of the horse. More often than not we were told that we had been examining a fit and healthy animal for the last hour. But these sessions were never a waste of time. After all, the amused staff argued, 'If you cannot recognise a healthy animal, how on earth will you recognise a sick one?' At the end of every tutorial we were always told to remember one thing; 'You won't always know the answer, but you can always use your common sense.'

Soon I would have those magical letters after my name, BVSc MRCVS, and I would be looking for a job. We started to look seriously at the job adverts in the vets' weekly journal, the *Veterinary Record*. It is difficult to believe now that so many job advertisers stated that a married man was preferred. This discrimination would certainly be frowned on today. Anyway, luckily for me I was one of them. *Au revoir* Liverpool. Look out Cotswolds, here we come! We're on our way back, to stay this time ...

CHAPTER TWO

A VET ON ROUTE 66

In the summer of 1966, can you believe that anything could be more important than watching England winning the World Cup? In my case something could. The euphoria of being a newly-qualified vet was still burning and it was time to look for that job I had dreamed of for years. I scanned the back pages and the vacancy columns of the *Veterinary Record* each week. Most of the advertisements were still looking for that 'married man', which at that time was accepted as a normal preference, so at least I did not have to worry about getting wed in a hurry.

Actually, the advertiser was usually as interested in the spouse as the actual vet, for honourable reasons. Without mobile phones, somebody had to look after the practice phone, take out-of-hours calls, give reassuring advice to clients, and pass messages on to the farm where the husband was out calving the cow. Now who would be prepared to do that job for nothing? Right first time – the vet's wife, of course.

On a dreary wet August evening, Angela and I trundled along the road from Gloucester to Cirencester in our little grey Austin A30. For most of the journey the swishing windscreen wipers were working overtime. We loved this car. A couple of years previously it had belonged to a Liverpool solicitor. It wasn't a car you usually associated with solicitors, but when he advertised it in the *Liverpool Echo*, one hoped he was on the brink of promotion and not desperation. He drove it to our Liverpool flat in Brookdale Road one misty November evening, and my pre-sales inspection was carried out with a torch under the light of a street lamp. I do appreciate that the RAC would have suggested a more cautious time and place. But it did belong to a solicitor and, fortunately, he was an honest one.

His reassurances regarding the car, care and reliability were backed up by bundles of garage service bills. We shook hands and I happily parted with £100 of my hard-earned cash. We knew it was money well spent and the next few days were spent polishing, lubricating and adding every affordable additive to the water coolant, the oil and fuel.

The regard was reciprocal. In the worst of weathers, even on those occasions when the car was partly buried in snow, the little banger always fired first time when you turned the key. But enough about cars! Angela and I were on our way to our *second* interview.

The first one had been held in the picturesque Cotswold village of Winchcombe, where the local community have had pride in their Sudeley Castle, steeped in royal history, for centuries. It was a popular holiday home for Henry VIII and Anne Boleyn, where he enjoyed the hunting in the area and the hospitality that Sudeley offered. In recent times, for better or for worse, the village has become famous as a centre of nuptial activities for rich actresses and their pop star entourage. I don't suppose Henry would have been too concerned about pre-nuptial agreements. He seemed to have his own ideas on how marriage problems should be settled.

That particular interview had gone quite well, but it had gone on for a long time. Angela was at one stage left with the principal's better half while he and I made off to his surgery, which was in a delightful position in the main village square. By strange coincidence it happened to be the start of surgery consulting time and the first customers of the day were waiting at the door. The patient was a small Dachshund that had been under treatment for a few weeks. I was introduced to the owner and Mr White, the vet, suggested to his client that it was an ideal opportunity for Mr Smith to take a look at Jasper, the apprehensive-looking dog. I had never heard of an interview where the applicant actually got involved in ongoing cases, but it was, I supposed, a chance to demonstrate what I knew. I was conscious of Mr White taking notes on a clipboard he had brought with him from the house.

With an attempt at some sort of bedside manner I gave Jasper a quick once-over before pushing a thermometer into his rear end. It was 102.5°F, a neither here nor there temperature, though perhaps my insertion technique had been enough to raise his temperature a little. The recent history of any case in diagnosis is critically important, but in this instance everything I asked seemed to be answered reluctantly. It quickly became clear that all my questions had been asked before, perhaps many times over. Jasper's submandibular lymph glands were enlarged, as were the prescapular glands, and there was evidence of a much more widespread lymphatic system involvement.

Even as a newly qualified vet I knew this was likely to be a very serious problem. What on earth was I supposed to tell the client? What was I doing on this side of the consulting table at an interview anyway? Was I supposed to be demonstrating to Mr White and Jasper's owner that I had been trained to examine an animal competently? Or was the principal looking for a second opinion, or just anybody's opinion?

Eventually we returned to Mr White's house, the clipboard tucked firmly under his arm. After five hours, with Mr White still making notes on us, we excused ourselves. We dived into our trusty little A30 and headed back to Hucclecote as fast as the Austin would take us. A few days later I received a kind letter and the offer of a job in Winchcombe. With every respect and consideration, I declined it.

This particular evening our destination was Crudwell. This village, between Cirencester and Malmesbury, is probably better known today than it was in the 1960s, both as a tourist attraction and now a dormitory for Cirencester and beyond. The population has doubled, and the village has grown in size, but it still has the old-world charm that we enjoyed when we were younger. The box number in the advertisement to which I had replied described the practice as being on the Wiltshire/Gloucestershire border, and it was looking for a young vet with a minimum of one year's experience. 'Good working conditions' were offered, and 'salary commensurate with experience'. I had no experience whatsoever to offer, but as I philosophically (though slightly nervously) uttered to Angela en route, 'Well, nothing ventured, nothing gained'.

We sped out of Cirencester on the road to Tetbury and quite soon turned sharp left, hoping that our intention had been made clear to all other road users in the vicinity by the flick of the dashboard switch and the lifting of a short amber arm from somewhere on the nearside body of the car. The little 'signal trafficator' was not always obvious to other drivers and the basic manoeuvre of turning left or right frequently led to some hairy moments and the blaring of horns from all directions. It was only a short time before flashing light indicators were mandatory on all cars – fortunately before road rage had evolved.

We knew that our left turn would soon bring us to Crudwell, which we could see on our tattered road atlas was somewhere between Kemble and Malmesbury. The rain had stopped by the time we reached the semi-detached farmhouse where ex-Army Major Hubert Leslie Evans lived. We walked up the muddy path to the small green door, which opened before we had time to knock on it. I should say here that few people referred to Mr Evans as Hubert. Some of his friends called him Hugh, but most of the clients, and just about everyone else, called him Taff. Hugh held out a large chubby hand and invited us into his front room. He appeared to be a charming, well-built jovial Welshman in his mid-forties who asked us to be seated and offered us a cup of tea. We chatted mainly about my recent college history and Mr Evans told us about his practice – which was mainly agricultural – his ambitions and the reason for the vacancy. He let us know that he had already interviewed many candidates for the job but had not considered any of them suitable. I wondered what he must be thinking of me and my lack of experience, but we seemed to get on well. At times he became a little excited, particularly when I asked a technical question or something resembling one, and he began to stammer and stutter. He gave the impression of being a lonely bachelor and there appeared to be no end to his generosity. After an hour or so, Taff exclaimed he would be delighted if we joined his practice.

It was customary at the time for most practices to provide rented accommodation for the assistants, usually a flat for the single vet or a house for that married man. To make us feel 'really comfortable and at home' Taff had promised to go a step further and buy land from his farmer neighbour and build a bungalow for us, which he hoped would encourage us to have a long association with the practice. While he was organising all of this he wondered if we wouldn't mind living in the farmhouse he had recently bought across the fields. It was aptly named Odd Farm. This was to be the site of his dream. This was where he would build his veterinary hospital, complete with decorative hanging baskets. It seemed a little odd to us that these should be an item of priority at this stage. As we were shown around the musty old house my wife frequently glanced at me apprehensively.

'Bet she wishes she was back in our Liverpool flat', I muttered to myself as Taff rambled on. He would not have noticed; he was too anxious to tell us how convenient and sensible it would be having a vet living next door to the hospital.

'It is a bit damp in this house, Mr Evans', I remarked as politely as possible, looking at the wallpaper peeling off the walls in strips.

'Oh, that's nothing to worry about', he replied in his prominent Welsh accent. 'Just where there's been nobody living here for a few months. It will soon dry out.'

We were not really convinced by his reassuring words. He must have been desperate for me to take the job. He sensed our reservations and before we left him that evening he had agreed to sell all the property in the back of beyond and buy another that he had his eye on in the village which would be just as suitable for his hospital. In the meantime he would look for a smaller, warmer, drier place for us to live, just until our bungalow was built of course. We drove home feeling that we had truly fallen on our feet. It would not be long before we discovered that the reality was a little different from the rosy picture painted at the time of our meeting.

We arranged to take up the post two weeks later. Taff hinted at one stage that it would be quite in order to leave it for a couple of months before making a start, and perhaps we should take a holiday first. The reason for this thoughtful gesture was not so much that time was required to organise the new assistant's accommodation, but rather to organise his assistants. I had made it clear that with hardly two halfpennies to rub together I needed to start work without delay. This caused a dilemma.

The present assistant, John Bourne, was leaving the practice to take up a teaching post at the School of Veterinary Science at Bristol University. He was a very accomplished vet on whom Taff had come to rely for the last six years, particularly with regard to surgical cases and difficult clients. In other words, and to be more precise, the practice revolved around his able assistant. When John gave in his notice and explained what his intentions were, Taff hit the roof, panic probably being high on his list of emotions.

'If you are going to Bristol, it's up to the university to find me a replacement', he demanded, 'and I want six months' notice at least.'

That was asking a lot even in the 1960s.

It would be ungracious to suggest that as a result of our interview he went cap in hand to John, but despite all that had been said, Taff did meekly ask if he would consider leaving at the end of the month. A compromise was reached and for a month or so the practice had two assistants. In hindsight, for a new graduate with no experience, things worked out very well. John was a natural teacher and for my first few weeks in practice I had my own personal tutor, who frequently reminded me that 'the day you qualify is the day you start to learn'. I must have repeated those words on innumerable occasions to students and newly qualified vets over the years.

The two weeks that followed the interview went quickly. Each day we waited in vain for a note in the post telling us that Mr Evans had found one dry place for us to live in Crudwell village. With just a few days to go before the starting date I telephoned him for a progress report. I left the smoky red telephone box feeling rather down. Clearly he had not done anything at all about our accomodation, and I would have to pass on the disappointing news to Angela.

'Would we mind moving into Odd Farm just for a short time?' he had pleaded.

We dreaded the thought of it, but at this late stage our options were limited. We could with good reason let him know that we had changed our minds about taking up the position, or we could grin and bear it and move into the dilapidated farmhouse. We desperately needed work and so we chose the latter.

Angela made a few rooms look homely during our first weekend. Although it was early autumn we lit fires to reduce the level of humidity in the place. She put up kitchen, bedroom and lounge curtains even though it was difficult to imagine anyone looking in when you are in the middle of nowhere. We put light bulbs in every room. Whoever was last out had taken all the bulbs with them.

On our first Sunday evening we were pleased to spot some car headlights approaching across the fields and wondered who our visitor might be. Taff alighted from his Cortina Estate and we naturally assumed the principal of the practice was paying us a courtesy visit to wish us good luck at the start of a successful career. In the twenty minutes he spent with us it became clear that thoughts of our success and good fortune was clearly not on his mind. By now we were no longer surprised that he failed to mention an early move to somewhere a little more comfortable. Instead he had come with an astonishing suggestion.

'I think it would be a good idea you know, Ivor, if you were on duty every night for the first month so that you can get to know where the farms are.'

'In the dark?' I thought to myself. Grudgingly I acknowledged his request, knowing that it was probably not wise to get on the wrong side of the boss at this stage.

The next morning I jumped into the Austin and drove to Taff's house. After a tedious hour spent in his kitchen listening to what seemed idle telephone chat to all and sundry he took me to his office and introduced me to his secretary/book keeper Mrs Edwards, a local middle-aged lady who welcomed me to the practice. The office was actually an ancient holiday caravan sited at the front of the house.

Taff clearly enjoyed farming. Between the caravan and the lane was a group of young cattle in one side of an enclosure, and a number of sows with their litters on the other. Several young pigs were wandering around. I was surprised to see that the animals were covered in mud and most of the calves were more than ankle-deep in mire. It had been a wet summer and it was boggy ground, but I did not feel it was my business to question the husbandry further.

I asked about a calf that was alone in one of the pens.

'Oh that one's been lame for a day or so, Ivor. You might like to have a look at him when we get back later?' It wasn't until the following day that I had an opportunity to examine this calf. A day later I was treating it for a limb fracture. How the calf suffered a broken leg we shall never know.

My first morning, and most of that week, I spent being chauffeured by my boss from farm to farm and being introduced to clients. An often-stuttering Taff explained that I was the veterinary replacement for John, who would be leaving the practice shortly. John was highly thought of by the farmers and I became accustomed to watching their faces drop at the news and suffering the comment, 'He'll be a hard act to follow', or similar sentiments. It tested my confidence to the limit and I began to wonder if I should ever have accepted the job.

We arrived back at the office for a lunchtime break early in the afternoon. I knew Angela would be waiting at home eager to hear how I had enjoyed my first morning in practice, but I was surprised to find her waiting outside the back door of the house. She looked anxious.

'Ive, I can't go back into that house, there are mice everywhere!'

I opened the back door and walked cautiously across the stone floor. She was not exaggerating; I met several in the first minute. There was not a room in the house they were not occupying. Clearly the warmth and smell of good cooking had been enough to entice them out, or in. We decided to skip lunch and made a beeline for the largest ironmonger in Cirencester.

'Yes sir', the shop assistant replied to my query, 'we do have mousetraps. How many would you like?'

'That's great; I'll take all of them!' We left with twenty traps and without delay positioned them strategically around the house. The traps snapped at frequent intervals and were reset. We lay in bed that night listening to the sound of traps going off in distant rooms as the mice were caught.

'God, I hope we don't hear them go off in here', Ange said as she buried her head under the sheets. At 6 o'clock the next morning I quietly slipped out of bed and crept downstairs carrying two traps from the bedroom that needed resetting.

Later that morning I reported for duty at the caravan at 8.30 sharp. A plague of mice was not something Taff was particularly interested in, but already we had a further complaint. In some places the walls were drying out and in other places they were getting wetter, particularly at floor level.

'Just a matter of time before it all dries out', he remarked philosophically after a two-minute inspection and without applying much logic. At the end of the week I insisted on a further inspection as in some areas the plaster was so soggy it was in danger of falling off the walls. For the first time he looked a little concerned and agreed there might be a problem.

'I'll get my builder to have a look at it next week', he said, reassuringly.

Despite our roaring fires the walls deteriorated over the next few days. Eventually the builder arrived and pulled up the floor in the lounge. He must have thought he had found a lake. For some reason every drop of water from the bathroom discharged straight under the floorboards, and we were adding to the deluge by at least two bathfuls a day.

At the end of my first week I could look back with some satisfaction. I had spent much time with John and gained a lot of practical experience. Angela and I quickly started to enjoy Crudwell life and began to appreciate the company of our neighbours. The farm closest to our house was run by Stanley Baldwin and his wife. They milked a small herd of about thirty cows and supplied us with milk, eggs and, more importantly, gossip. The couple were in their mid-fifties and struggled to adapt to the changes in lifestyle that the 1960s had brought about. The first time Angela collected milk from his little dairy, Stanley was delighted to demonstrate his recently installed lighting system in the cowshed. He seemed to believe it was almost a miracle that he could now switch off the lights from either end of the shed on his way out, no matter which end they had been switched on.

Stanley's driving was best suited to deserted country lanes. Motorways were a new experience and he clearly had difficulty coming to terms with a new set of rules of the road. He generously offered to take Angela and his wife on a trip to look at the recently constructed Severn Road Bridge. Having completed the mission Stanley felt that it was rather a waste of time and petrol to continue along the motorway, but unable to spot a turning he commenced to manoeuvre to the outside lane in order to do a U-turn. Angela's yells from the rear made him realise he might perhaps be doing something wrong. After tactfully bringing him up to date with the new rules, he grudgingly continued in the same direction.

Stanley was a chap you could not be cross with for long. He just seemed to be someone who was unaware that rules applied in life, even when they were unwritten. I am sure it never occurred to him that sometimes his veterinary neighbour might not be on duty and would really appreciate some sleep, especially at 5 o'clock in the morning. One chilly November morning we were woken by the unusual sound of objects hitting our bedroom window and muffled noises coming from below. We recognised Stanley's voice calling out, 'Mr Smith, Mr Smith'.

I opened the window as he prepared to chuck his next handful of gravel in my direction. I suspect that he often communicated in this manner, but perhaps only in times of necessity. Needless to say, Stanley had yet to delve into the advantages of being on the telephone.

'Can you come and see my cow? I've just found her down on the ground and I think she's got a touch of milk fever.'

'Certainly', I answered, trying to sound cheerful and disguise the 'first thing in the morning' look my wife insists that I have.

'Be with you in a few minutes', I shouted down, as I fumbled for my jeans.

Half an hour later, Stanley's freshly calved cow had been given a large intravenous dose of calcium and was back on her feet. Hypocalcaemia, or milk fever, is a potentially life-threatening illness, and was, and still is, a very simple and satisfying problem to treat. He was grateful for my promptness, and in return I was grateful to him for including Angela in their weekly shopping trip to Cirencester.

The shopping ritual began early each Friday morning when Stanley and his wife were picked up by Mr and Mrs Keen – Ivy and Percy – in their immaculate Jaguar. Friday was really the only time this beautiful car saw the light of day. Behind the powerful engine lay a spacious leather interior. Anything smaller and Ivy would have been unable to get in. She was a rotund lady, but kind and always jovial. Each week Angela squeezed in with the ladies and caught up on the village gossip. We were always intrigued to hear what Taff had been up to in recent days that we had not heard about, and not surprisingly Taff was the centre of the conversation within minutes. There never was a dull moment with Taff.

It was the Keens' misfortune to be living in the other half of the semi-detached farmhouse to Taff. I do not know how this arrangement came about but we knew from experience how persuasive he could be.

We began to wonder what had become of the person we had met at our interview. This one certainly had a short fuse and, living next door, Mrs Keen saw the worst of his temper all too often. One morning, from her window, she watched Taff enter his caravan office to speak to a farmer client on the phone. As he left and stepped down the few steps, the telephone rang again. For some reason he showed his irritation by slamming the caravan door hard enough for it to break the hinges. Mrs Keen watched in amazement as the pantomime was repeated, but when the telephone rang on the next occasion, the slamming of the door caused it to part company with the caravan and it fell to the ground.

On their way to Cirencester one Friday, Angela and the farmers' wives as usual swapped stories of their week's events, but it was of Mr Evans' tale that the majority in the car awaited news.

'You'll never guess what he did this week', Ivy began. All knew that anything was possible.

'Well, he was going out to feed his pigs with a bucket of meal in both his hands when the phone went. Mrs Edwards called from the caravan to say a farmer wanted to speak to him, and that it was urgent.' Ivy chuckled as everyone in the car waited to hear what was coming next.

'I can't come now. Can't you see I'm busy?' he shouted back.

'But he says it's very urgent and he must speak to you now', replied an anxious Mrs Edwards, wondering what the reaction would be. Taff's response was maniacal. The air turned blue as, among other things, he ranted about always being at the farmers' beck and call.

'I'd never heard words like it before', Ivy declared piously, 'so I told him to go and wash his mouth out with soap and water.' Mrs Keen must have rubbed salt into the wound, for Taff responded by throwing the buckets of pig food into the air. He was standing under a large apple tree.

'All the apples came down on his head!' roared Mrs Keen, her sides almost splitting.

The days and weeks went quickly, for me anyway. For most of the day Angela was home alone apart from the odd mouse for company. It was a lonely existence, which she frequently relieved by walking to one of the neighbouring farms for a chat.

We had another unusual neighbour. Across the fields, farmer Stanley's grounds adjoined RAF Kemble, which at this time was the base of the famous Red Arrows flying team. As the planes flew past, their wings tip to tip as they soared and dived, they provided us with unique entertainment. We were sure that Odd Farm was a marker for some of their dazzling practice runs. It was not unusual to see a couple of jets diving silently towards the farmhouse. If you missed them coming toward you, you certainly did not miss them leaving as they roared off into the distance. Even when Taff was not around there never seemed to be a dull moment.

The end of my first month in the job came and went. Things were not turning out as we had expected but I was beginning to gain that all-important experience. I particularly enjoyed the company of assistant John, with whom, in theory anyway, I was on a par. At my interview with Mr Evans I had eventually brought up the subject of money, an issue which appeared to be of more importance to me than to him. It transpired that the starting salary I had in mind was the amount he was paying John. He agreed to pay me the same without any negotiation at all. What a generous man, we thought.

There was a special sense of excitement carrying out night visits, albeit in the company of another vet. Usually we attended a cow having difficulty calving or down with milk fever, or calves with pneumonia, or a bitch having a problem whelping. Occasionally it was something a little different.

One evening John and I treated a herd of milking cows that had broken into a food store and eaten a huge amount of concentrated feed. This was a nightmare to treat, one of the problems being that usually you had no idea which animal had eaten what and how much. It was not simply a case of a herd of cows suffering from indigestion. The complications that could rapidly develop from gorging rich cereal food frequently led to fatalities.

Typically, when you arrived at a farm to treat such a case, you were greeted by a farmer in a state of shock and a herd with some of the cows looking normal and others staggering around the yard. Untreated, some of the cows would die as the contents of the stomach became increasingly more acidic: this acid corrosion resulting in stomach erosion. Treatment could involve performing rumenotomy, where surgery is carried out on the largest of the cow's stomachs and the food physically removed by hand. Most would receive large volumes of intravenous fluids. Some may not recover even with treatment and would need to be sent for emergency slaughter as quickly as possible. Deciding which receives treatment and which you slaughter is sometimes a very difficult choice.

As we drove back through the village, John suggested we called in at The Plough for a quick pint, which I was more than happy to agree to. As we walked across the road to the pub, John, whose thirst for knowledge and teaching was insatiable, asked with great interest what I had been taught at Liverpool about cereal over-eating in cattle. I knew that I was about to hear the latest research on the subject. We supped our pints and the viva continued. I remember those 'end of the day' occasions with pleasure. Perhaps we had discovered the true meaning of a 'thirst for knowledge'.

The Plough in the 1960s was a typical old-fashioned English village pub, attracting occasional visitors during the day, but acting mainly as the rendezvous for the locals at night. The darts board was in constant demand. The players may have been farm labourers by day but their mental arithmetic at night – as they calculated what was needed at the next throw – was astonishing. I often watched in amazement. Today it is still an appealing pub but it now has the added attraction of a fine restaurant. No doubt the business is run on more formal lines than forty years ago when we were customers. At closing time back then the front door was locked at 11 p.m., sometimes with the regulars on the inside, and drinking continued until everyone decided it was time to go home. On one occasion, allegedly, the local bobby knocked on the door late one night.

'If you're coming in', the landlady shouted, 'Put your bicycle round the back.'

It was the end of my first month in practice and for all the obvious reasons I looked forward to pay day. It is normal practice in most businesses to pay your staff for their efforts at the end of the month, or at least early the next. In Mr Evans' practice a cheque had still not materialised halfway through the second month and every daily request was met with a strange new reason for not paying. I gave in my notice and sure enough the next day the cheque appeared.

There was a repeat performance the following month, but on this occasion I was determined to leave the practice without further delay unless prompt payment was combined with an effort to move us out of the isolated, cold, damp farmhouse. A chilly Wiltshire winter was fast approaching. The end of the third month became the final demand. Things were beyond a joke and our sense of humour had evaporated.

Then, as unexpectedly as ever, Taff surprised everyone. At the 8.30 briefing one morning he was pleased to report that he had some pleasant news for me. Perhaps he was about to announce that he was going to pay me this month before I handed in my notice for the fourth time.

'I have decided to sell Odd Farm and I have bought a place in the village, Ivor, which I think would make a much better veterinary hospital', Taff pronounced. I looked for somewhere to sit before I fell down.

'I think you will be happier there as well', he added, more quietly. It sounded like a bit of an afterthought. His predictions were at least half right. I could not stop thinking how much he sounded like Aneurin Bevan giving a major parliamentary speech on profound social changes in the Valleys as he proudly rambled on. 'Wonder where the hanging baskets will go?' I thought. Hugh Evans finally had his veterinary dream, even if they did seem a little over-ambitious, and suddenly our world was much brighter, warmer and drier. We were on the move again.

CHAPTER THREE

IN AT THE DEEP END

The property Taff had bought in the centre of the picturesque village of Crudwell was, to be fair, an assistant's dream. Ridgeway Farm was to one side of the village green. By the 1960s the grounds of the farm had been incorporated into neighbouring farms and only the old farmhouse and outbuildings remained, on opposite sides of a gravel yard. For many years it was the base for a haulage company owned by the Carpenter family, who had now reached retirement age. In his usual fashion Taff had used charm and persuasion to do a deal with Mrs Carpenter, apparently, so they say, leaving her late one night mentally exhausted following a long-winded negotiating session. And by means fair or foul he had struck a bargain, which he told me included generously writing off her outstanding veterinary fees.

The house itself was very old indeed, probably dating back to the seventeenth century, and was believed to have once been used as a candle factory. Upstairs there was not a level floor in the place. It was an enjoyable place to make a home, and it had been sympathetically brought into the twentieth century by the installation of oil-fired central heating, which was more than a little welcome in December. Previous owners had fortunately retained its charm and sense of history but modern furniture blended in well and from time to time we bought items from the G–Plan range when there was something left over from the monthly payments on the cooker, washing machine and bed.

We had persuaded Mr Evans that his insistence on using the study in our house as the practice office was not a good idea. The thought of having to repair the hinges of our doors following an unwelcome telephone call was unimaginable, and, in any case, logic stipulated that the office should be inside the new hospital on the other side of the yard.

It was not long before the plans had been drawn up and proudly displayed to everyone. They were impressive. The large Cotswold-stone barn would house a reception area, a large waiting room, kennel rooms, operating theatres and most of the facilities found in a modern veterinary hospital. The building itself was big enough to include two apartments, one for Taff and a smaller one for his second assistant. To be charitable it was good forward planning, but even to an inexperienced young vet the project did not make good business sense. Clearly Taff's heart was ruling his head. Where was the money coming from to pay for all this?

Nevertheless the building work started and was completed in months. The standard of workmanship was remarkable. The building contractors were the Ball brothers from Tetbury. There seemed to be a brother for every trade that was needed to do the job. It was fascinating to watch the mason cutting the stones and the carpenter making joints in the timber with his ancient tools. Finally the brothers produced a sibling painter, or at least a cousin. The job was completed on time. This was a remarkable feat considering the number of times Taff decided he would prefer something to be in a different place.

I pulled into the yard one lunchtime at the end of my morning's rounds to find him standing outside admiring his new building, a slightly puzzled look on his face.

'Anything amiss, Mr Evans?' I asked.

'No, not really', he replied. 'I'm just wondering where to put the hooks for the hanging baskets.'

Taff at last had his hospital. Well, he had a building that he called a hospital, and up went the sign, 'Ridgeway Veterinary Hospital'. It all sounded very grand, but it was a very contentious thing to do. There existed a group of prominent practising veterinary surgeons at that time, who, with the blessing of our governing body, the Royal College of

Veterinary Surgeons, had formed a Veterinary Hospitals Association whose aim was to promote the highest standards of medical and surgical care for their patients. To qualify, and for the practice to be included on this list, an official inspection was required to ensure that the standards, with regard to facilities and trained staff, were maintained or existed in the first place.

No matter how good the intentions, an empty building naturally fell a little short of requirements. As regards trained staff we had Sheila, the daughter of a local farmer. She was very sweet and willing, but veterinary nursing was not her forte. She was employed to look after Taff's pigs and calves, which she did second to none. When asked by the vet, she held a dog correctly so that an intravenous injection could be given, but that was the full extent of her skills. If Mr Evans knew anything of these hospital regulations he chose simply to ignore them.

Like most vets at that time my boss was aware that there was a promising lucrative future in the care of pets that we refer to today as companion animals. Big oaks grow from small acorns and Taff was ready to plant. His choice of building, prior to his hospital, would be frowned upon by planners today. His one-room surgery was an outbuilding adjoining the Mayfield Hotel, whose restaurant featured in the *Good Food Guides* of the day. How he persuaded the hotel owners to let him do this is anyone's guess.

Taff delegated the running of the small animal side of the business to his assistant; in other words I carried out the surgeries. Initially these commenced at 2 p.m., which meant that on most days there was hardly time to swallow a lunchtime sandwich. But it was enjoyable and a good opportunity to meet and chat to local people. When things went well they went very well, but when they didn't, they could be horrific.

On one occasion in my first week a Mrs Jones came to the surgery with her daughter, Samantha. She was carrying every vet's nightmare, 'something in a cardboard box'. Soon all was revealed. Samantha whipped off the lid of the box to reveal two pet mice.

'It's just a quick routine visit, Mr Smith', Mrs Jones explained. 'My daughter wants to be sure they are fit and healthy and that she's doing all the right things.'

'They look fine to me, Mrs Jones, but I'll give them the once-over just to be sure', I answered confidently.

I swear the first mouse I lifted from that box was the most elusive that was ever born. He slipped from my hands and, as I tried to grab him, he dashed along the table. Sadly the table wasn't quite long enough and Samantha's pet fell headlong to the floor. I didn't have another chance to grab him before he disappeared through a gap between the floorboards. Mother and daughter looked stunned, but worse was to come. Shocked at having lost the first patient, nobody had noticed his pal climbing out of the cardboard box and charging down the table after him. Before I could catch him, he too had dived off the end and without further hesitation followed his mate through the floorboards. Well, in a situation like that what can you say?

I was more than sorry, naturally, but apologising to a hysterical young girl seemed a bit inadequate. Eventually, carrying their now empty box, they left the surgery in complete silence. I didn't feel they were impressed with my professional competence. I would have loved to suggest that the two mice, now nesting next door to a *cordon bleu* restaurant, would live happily ever after, but I did not think it would go down too well.

One aspect of my work that has given me immense satisfaction throughout my career has been performing surgical procedures. I was never happier than spending most of my day with a scalpel in one hand and forceps in the other. For whatever reason surgical work was not Taff's forte and I was grateful for the opportunity to tackle any such cases that came my way. I would have been happier and more confident if the practice had provided some of the surgical basics that were available at the time. I can imagine Mr Evans describing his operating theatre as minimalist, but by the end of most operations Heath-Robinson would have been more apt. A veterinary nurse trained in medical and surgical routines would have been a dream come true, but Sheila did her best and I instructed her step by step as we went along.

The old wooden operating-cum-examination table was scrubbed down, allowed to dry and the anaesthetised patient positioned on a clean blanket. The hair surrounding the surgical site was laboriously clipped away with scissors before Sheila scrubbed away at the exposed skin for a few minutes – following the scrubbing of her own hands for a bit longer to remove the remnants of her pig management duties. Under the circumstances we did quite well and I was usually happy with the outcome. Ingenuity and compromise were the orders of the day and we both managed to keep our sense of humour.

There were some farmers in the practice who, for one reason or another, refused to allow a new graduate anywhere near their livestock and it was a long time before I ventured on to the premises of Mr Burdon. At some stage in my first year he relented and I got on quite well with him after that, having recovered from the initial nervousness of meeting him, and I enjoyed going there. He was not only a successful dairy farmer but he also enjoyed a reputation for breeding winning racing greyhounds.

He also had another reputation: he frequently swore, but he swore like no one else I have met before or since. Whenever he got cross, which seemed to be most of the time, a tirade of expletives leapt forth. To say you had never heard anything like it would be a monumental understatement. It seemed impossible for him to express himself adequately, so the start of one known word would be added to the end of another and it sounded for all the world as though he were inventing his own vocabulary of imaginative profanities. Eventually, having shocked everyone within earshot, his wrath was overcome with mirth and he frequently ended up chuckling at his own theatricals.

One day when I was on the farm he asked if I had time to look at a lame greyhound that had suffered a foot injury during a recent race. The injury was a common one, 'a knocked-up toe', and before I had time to discuss any treatment options, he said, 'I don't suppose you've taken a toe off before, have you?' From his body language on this occasion he seemed to know that I had not and was thus giving me the opportunity to operate on this one. It was a procedure that was frequently carried out to treat this condition and in the hands of an experienced surgeon was little more than routine. But nothing could be described as routine in our surgery and for me at the time this was major surgery. To add spice to the occasion Mr Burdon insisted on being present throughout. I have never been sure whether he wanted to assess my surgical skills or be certain I removed the right toe.

The heavily sedated greyhound was positioned on a clean blanket and the foot prepared for surgery. Wisely I chose not to administer a general anaesthetic, which at that time would have been a long-acting intravenous barbiturate. Greyhounds are notorious for reacting adversely to generals, and an anaesthetic emergency was the last thing I needed with this audience. Movement of the patient without one could be a problem, but with Sheila's weight bearing down on the dog this was reduced to a minimum. I had confidence in the tourniquet that she had applied tightly to the leg to control haemorrhage should I fail to find and ligate the digital blood vessels.

I tried to ignore Mr Burdon's presence and what he might be thinking as I made a Y-shaped incision over the toe and began the dissection. I would have liked to have watched the anxious expression on his face as blood oozed from the wound, but his cap was pulled down menacingly over his eyes. Throughout the operation he remained remarkably silent.

It was not a long operation. I clamped and tied off the small artery and toe veins, disarticulated the damaged toe joint to complete the amputation, and stitched up. We applied a pressure bandage and the job was done. Mr Burdon lifted his sleepy greyhound almost affectionately and placed him gently on hessian sacks in the back of an old van. The operation had gone well and I felt he was satisfied and grateful, and although he said little he did manage a few choice words. Mr Burdon was probably approaching fifty at the time and his charming wife well into her forties. They had several children who were in their late teens and I suspect he was more than a little surprised when he discovered that Mrs Burdon was expecting another. No doubt he had a few choice words on that occassion.

For reasons known only to himself, Mr Evans opened a branch surgery behind the windows of a little shop on the High Street at Cricklade, another pretty Cotswold village about 7 miles from Cirencester. Professional attendance was limited to one hour per week on a Thursday evening and, not surprisingly, the surgery was run by the vet assistant. I suppose you could argue that any service is better than none and for some it avoided the inconvenience of travelling to Cirencester, Lechlade or one of the other nearby Cotswold villages. Facilities were, by any stretch of the imagination, a bit spartan. The examination table was the old shop counter. The original shop owner lived in rooms at the back, and at 6.30 p.m. always provided a large china bowl of hot water as a hand wash, and a towel. Needless to say after an hour it was cold and murky and looked like a big bowl of cold soup. Having seen perhaps up to half a dozen patients, I closed the shop at around 8 o'clock and drove home as fast as I could. It was by rota off-duty time and I looked forward to at least a short evening at home. There was no need to look at my watch. In the background I had been listening all night to the landlady's television.

One Thursday night I had done surgery to the accompaniment of Terry Wogan and his commentary on the Eurovision Song Contest. In 1967 it was one of the television highlights of the year and on this occasion a barefoot Sandie Shaw was our great hope. I normally left the surgery to the sound of music, and on this particular night it was 'Puppet on a String', which won the competition. Those were the good old days when England had not upset enough people to be awarded 'nul points'.

At the start of each month Taff produced the vets' duty rota. This was an important document. It was the only indication I had of knowing whether I was on duty on a Monday, Tuesday or any other night of the week. It was a certainty that the following week the off-duty nights would be different. We wondered at first what the logic behind his thinking was until we realised that he was working backwards. He filled in the nights he wanted to socialise and gave his recovery nights to me.

Our social life had been on hold for a few months since we left Liverpool. Things improved rapidly after we moved to Crudwell. Our house was close to the main road through the village and consequently there was always activity of some kind. In some way or other most of the traffic, tractors, trailers and cattle lorries that hurtled past was related to farming. Our immediate neighbours kept the post office next door and we soon became friends with them and the young local couple beyond them. It was lovely having someone to chat to in the day and to pop down to the pub with for a quick pint in the evening. Removing the practice from my mind for any length of time was a different matter.

Eight-thirty each morning arrived all too quickly. Taff sorted out the morning calls and off we went in different directions. That was the usual plan, but one day things went disastrously wrong on the road. I had spent my morning on the east side of the practice while Mr Evans had gone west. To finish my calls I slipped back to a farm to revisit a cow with a severe mastitis that I had seen the day before, to ensure she was responding to the antibiotic treatment I had given her.

It was a beautiful day as I travelled west, unknowingly on a collision course with Taff, who was now returning home travelling east. Half a mile from the practice, along a quiet narrow road, I spotted a large grey car approaching and slowed to allow each of us ample time to move to the nearside of the lane to pass comfortably. This simple manoeuvre did, however, depend on each driver being aware of the other being there, and I started to have my doubts. As the vehicles got closer it became obvious that the driver of the approaching car hadn't seen me, and to my horror I recognised the unmistakable face of my boss. I first saw the profile of his face. He was looking sideways, admiring the hedgerow and whistling the time away. I stared in disbelief and in a desperate last measure I leaned heavily on my car horn. Suddenly, Taff's large Cortina Estate started to skid and judder and jump towards me as he stood on his brakes. I waited for the inevitable impact. Following the sound of bending metal and breaking glass things were quiet again for a moment. Taff bashed the inside of his car a few times to release the jammed door and struggled out while the air around him turned blue.

Following a lecture on the need to drive with extreme care on country roads he disappeared down the lane towards the practice to telephone our local garage, leaving me with two cars blocking the road and warning oncoming traffic of an obstruction. With their wheels almost in the ditch it was just possible for other vehicles to squeeze by. At 8.30 the next morning the lecture on safe driving continued. To emphasise his concern regarding road safety, later that week Taff installed a roadside mirror at the end of his drive to warn him of unseen approaching traffic. A wise move, but it seemed to have little relevance to not looking where you are going. I decided not to comment.

With cars repaired I was free again to enjoy my job and the beautiful Cotswold countryside. One of my favourite destinations was the drive to the old rural estates of Lord Sam Vestey at Stowell Park, tucked away about 9 miles from Cirencester. Although I rarely had the opportunity to meet his young lordship, who was twenty-one at the time, it was a pleasure to work with his farm staff. A large number of the chaps I met had worked on the estate all their lives and were very good stockmen. Most understood my lack of experience but appreciated the skills and knowledge that I did have.

I have always enjoyed driving and the only time I ever became frustrated were those odd occasions when I arrived back home only for Angela to say that the farm manager had rung to ask me to pop back to look at another sheep or steer in trouble. 'Popping back' was another 30-odd-mile round trip. Three cheers for today's mobile phone.

Emergency cases were not few and far between. With so many animals there was always the odd steer or heifer with the rapid onset of a severe respiratory infection, or cattle or sheep developing a sudden painful lameness. From time to time there was the satisfaction of helping a struggling heifer in labour and delivering an oversize calf. A great deal of the work was routine and there was plenty of it. Castrating and disbudding young calves was one of these procedures. It could become a little monotonous and thus was often a task that, unsurprisingly, was normally carried out by the assistant vet. Disbudding involved handling the calves on two occasions. To deal with the large number of calves, sometimes fifty or more in one session, the animals were run through a small calf-size cattle crush. They were injected with a local anaesthetic to freeze the area of the small horn buds on their heads, and then run through the crush again to remove the buds by burning them off with a red-hot iron. This may sound horrific but done correctly the procedure is painless.

On one of the estate's farms, I must have dealt with hundreds of calves in this manner and one of my regular helpers was an old weather-beaten stockman named Harry, although of course most called him 'Arry. He was at least seventy and very fit and agile for his years. He probably enjoyed a pint but I knew he was not a smoker, and he always liked a chat. At this time it seemed as though everyone was a smoker, including me. At the end of my first calf disbudding session there, having packed the kit back in the car, I lit up and offered 'Arry a cigarette.

'No thanks, son', he said. 'Don't touch 'em these days. 'Aven't 'ad a fag now since I 'ad bronchitis in the twenties.'

'That's a long time ago, 'Arry; do you ever feel like one?' I asked.

'Yeah, I do', he replied, 'Every bloody day of my life for the last forty years.'

Disbudding some frisky calves on one occasion, 'Arry started to talk about the hot iron I was using, which was heated from the gas in a portable Calor gas cylinder.

'Better than the way we used to do it', he reminisced. 'We used to burn a fire and when it was red hot we'd stick the irons in the fire. Well yer Mr Evans was 'ere one day doing the calves and nothing seemed to go right, and he started shouting and bawling at everybody. Things went from bad to worse and we couldn't get the irons 'ot enough and he was taking so long the anaesthetic started to wear off and that made things worse. I don't know who he thought he was talking to, but he called us everything you can imagine', related 'Arry at length.

'I couldn't stand any more, so when he shouted for another iron that I'd only just stuck in the fire, and he told me how useless I was, I thought I'd give 'im something to shout about, so I gave 'im the hot end first', 'Arry chuckled. I winced, but I had to smile secretly at what might have followed. I could see that iron disappearing across the field.

I probably disbudded and castrated more than my fair share of calves, as practice assistants probably still do today, but it gave me the chance to meet the farmers in the area so that it didn't come as too much of a shock when I turned up at their farm at night to calve their cow. The dairy cow was the most important animal in the area. Most of my days were spent attending her ailments. If she had recently calved and was ill, I usually managed to remember my three Ms. There was an odds-on chance that she was probably suffering from mastitis, metritis or milk fever. Our Liverpool lecturers who taught us clinical medicine emphasized the importance of this simplicity and it was particularly reassuring on those occasions when at first sight you had no idea what was wrong with her, and it often led to the right diagnosis.

As the months went by I grew in confidence and increasingly enjoyed the work. Occasionally I examined a cow with a 'left displaced abomasum'. In very simple terms this meant that one of the cow's complicated four-stomach structure had decided to travel from its normal position on the right of the midline to somewhere on the left. These normally high-yielding cows became inappetent and their inadequate food intake resulted in a great loss in milk production. Diagnosis was not rocket science. Having eliminated other possibilities, with your ear, or preferably your stethoscope, pressed close to the cow's left flank, palpating the abdomen with your fist produced the wonderful chimes of the wandering stomach. I found it was one of those conditions where in fact you could hear more without the stethoscope. Unfortunately, some of the cows you listened to had lice. At the end of the day my first priority when I arrived home was to wash my hair in an insecticidal shampoo. Taking your patient's parasites home with you was an occupational hazard.

We had been taught various surgical techniques at Vet School to correct the condition but I was impressed by the one that my predecessor, John, had taught me. No doubt many aspects of our procedure would be frowned upon today. The farmer collected a drench from the surgery containing the anaesthetic chloral hydrate that I had prepared in advance. When I arrived at the farm the farmer would have drenched the cow an hour or so previously and she would be about to collapse on a deep bed of straw. The anaesthetised animal was propped on her back with straw bales and prepared for surgery. An incision was made into the abdomen; the aberrant stomach identified, moved to its correct position and surgically fixed to ensure that it stayed in place. The success rate was high and it was satisfying to see that cow feeding well and in excellent production a few weeks later. My first two or three cases were weekend occasions arranged to allow John to be away from the Bristol Vet School for the day and it was a joint effort. They all survived the operation. Initially, John did the surgery as far as the closure of the abdomen. The next part, the long boring bit, was the closing of the cow's musculature and skin. That was my job. I was grateful for John's time and it was not long before I was doing this operation alone on any old day of the week.

It did not take long to realise that in your early days in farm practice your reputation with local farmers often depended on your ability to calve a cow. You were frequently on the farm for several hours giving the farmer the chance to find out your life history, what you knew and what you didn't. Most calvings, especially the difficult ones, always seemed to occur late at night or very early in the morning. I soon learned to anticipate how difficult the task might be by the tone of voice on the end of the telephone. Some farmers always erred on the side of caution and at the first sign of anything unusual picked up the phone. The amount of assistance these cows required was usually minimal and a vaginal examination told you immediately that all was well and perhaps all that was needed was a little more time.

'Sometimes', John said, with tongue in cheek, 'you need to put your hand against the calf's head to stop them coming out too quickly or it might look as though you weren't really needed.'

But for every straightforward calving, there were twenty cases where you really earned your money. This was often true with the large unit where there was often an experienced farm manager who had received some formal instruction on bovine obstetrical problems at an agricultural college. When they rang you could bet problems lay ahead. Sometimes it would have been better if they had admitted defeat and called you sooner. This delay frequently meant the difference between delivering a live calf or a dead one.

Within minutes of examining the patient a plan of action can usually be determined. The calf may have one front leg pointing in the wrong direction, or both, or the head is twisted back, or the whole calf is trying to come out backwards. The name of the game was to try to rearrange the limbs in the quickest time with as little harm to the cow as possible. This was usually performed with the aid of soft ropes, a lot of soapsuds, and as much strength as your arms could muster. Once the calf was in the correct position for delivery, with ropes attached to the forelimbs and sometimes the head as well, traction was applied and the calf was pulled into its new world. Naturally, for humane reasons, there was a limit to how much traction could be applied to the ropes in attempting to extract a particularly large calf. The rule of thumb that we were taught at Vet School was that if no progress had been made after twenty minutes with two strong men on each rope, a caesarean operation should be performed.

Often, the difficulty was finding four strong men when you needed them. This was the situation one Saturday evening at a farm near Siddington, a small village near Cirencester. I knew the farm staff well and I was always happy to work with Sid and Joe, a couple of salt-of-the-earth brothers who were always helpful and obliging when I was at the farm carrying out routine work. Sid was ready to greet me when I arrived at about 10 o'clock, armed with the obligatory bucket of hot water, soap and towel. I was soon able to tell him that the cow he was worried about would calve without too much trouble but because of his size – the odds were that it was a bull calf – the calf would need a bit of a pull to deliver him. I explained that we would need a bit more manpower to do the job. Within minutes Sid had located Joe. They were lovely guys but with every respect, their combined stature did not really add up to one strong man. After five minutes of sibling traction, it became clear that the calf was quite happy to remain where he was, immersed in his mother's warm fluids.

'I think we are likely to need a little more help, Sid', I tactfully suggested. 'Is there anyone else around tonight?'

'I'll go and see who is about Mr Smith', he answered, almost apologetically. Within minutes he had produced Albert, who was now retired but had worked on the farm all his life. I do not doubt that in his youth he had been the athletic saviour of many calves, but that was clearly many years ago. The brothers took one rope and Albert the other. The calf remained stationary, but I was sure that with a reasonable pull it could be safely delivered. I was as much concerned about Albert's wellbeing as the calf's, because he was puffing and panting alarmingly.

'Do you think you could find any other volunteers, chaps?'

'Not easy at this time on a Saturday, Mr Smith – they're all down the pub. But we'll have a go.'

The brothers disappeared and I whiled away the minutes with Albert chatting about farming tales in the area over the last century, while at the same time lubricating the calf and the walls of the encapsulating uterus with bubbly soapsuds, until we heard voices in the distance. The many voices seemed to be part of a crowd. Then Sid appeared at the entrance to the barn with his followers. He must have emptied the pub and all the locals had turned up to calve the cow. They swarmed in and I found myself at the back of the shed some distance from my patient. There were so many inebriated lads present that the ropes weren't long enough to take them all. Eventually, with something resembling the regional tug-of-war championships, I gave the order to pull. The calf shot out like a cork from a bottle. Nestled on a bed of deep straw, he was content to be admired by the customers of his village local.

It is strange how from one generation to the next so much of country life revolves around two institutions: the church and the village pub. The village of Crudwell was no different. If the major part of village life did officially revolve around All Saints' Church, a little was certainly taken up at the local pub. In our case it was The Plough, which was opposite the church and handy for the vicar to pop in and chat to his parishioners. It was also a popular venue for entertaining visiting vet college and old school pals, whom we were always pleased to see.

My principal's reputation preceded him and shortly after their arrival my pals would ask, 'What's Taffy been up to recently?' They were rarely disappointed. Hardly a week went by without a calamity of some description.

There was a memorable occasion when, for once, my boss was not involved. The Beddises were staying with us for the weekend. We had known Colin and Rene, who both proudly originated from the Forest of Dean, since schooldays. On Saturday night Colin and I left our wives to chat at home while we popped along the road for a quick one at The Plough. Colin had suggested going for a cross-country run the following morning. He was a very good athlete, and after our third pint I had agreed to go with him. We continued to put the world to rights and at closing time made our way back to Ridgeway House.

At 9 o'clock on Sunday morning we foundourselves duly jogging along country lanes. It was a long time since I had done any running, recreational anyway, but I was enjoying it and the first mile went well. As the morning went on the miles seemed to get longer and when we eventually arrived back in Crudwell, we re-hydrated ourselves and took a bath. I took to my bed and Colin took to the road in his car to check how far we had run. He was a director in a firm of builders, and I guess this was the sort of thing that interested surveyors. It has been easy to remember just how far we did run that morning. For every pint we had the night before we had run a mile. It had been a seven-mile run. It is hard to believe that fate would take a wicked turn. Less than a year later Colin developed a rare but serious illness and died within weeks of its onset. Rene has remained a close friend and we often look back on those hilarious days with fondness. Today she is able to enjoy her grandchildren. Colin lived just long enough to enjoy his own daughter for a few short months.

We quickly became friends with local villagers and I particularly enjoyed the company of the Pettifer family. Stephen, or Steffy as he was known locally, was an elderly retired veterinary surgeon who a decade before had been the principal of the Crudwell practice. It was fascinating to swap veterinary anecdotes with him. He was a descendant of Thomas Pettifer, whose family had been manufacturing horse and farm animal medicines since 1867. How effective they all were I cannot say. The labels on some of the bottles I saw suggested that they cured most things, but the proof of the pudding was in the eating, or, in most cases, the forcible drenching. The various medicines all seemed to have one thing in common: their taste and smell was horrendous, and if I was the sick beast I would want to get better quickly before I got a second dose.

These were the days before 24-hour news television but we were now at the start of the era of seeing news as it happened. The black and white images of current tragedies, like the schoolchildren of Aberfan buried under a mountain of sliding coal, will forever be impressed on my mind. The only news is bad news it seemed and that fatal landslide happened to be an interlude from the horrors of the war in Vietnam. Each night you switched on the TV there was a news item from the front line and a report on the latest fighting, usually brought to you by a bullet-ducking BBC reporter. One brave reporter happened to be Julian Pettifer, the son of my friend Stephen.

'When he's home next I'll make sure you'll meet him', Steffy said one evening over a pint in The Plough. True to his word, that Christmas I did.

If you were regularly on that little television screen in the 1960s everyone believed you must be a really eminent person, and usually you were. Today it seems that if you have been on television on more than one occasion you must be a celebrity, and usually you are not. When Steffy and Julian came to visit, the initial meeting was an odd experience. We saw him each night reporting the latest news from the war zone, and when we first saw him walking down our garden path it felt as if we were being visited by an old friend that we knew well. Of course he didn't know us from Adam, but a couple of glasses of sherry broke the ice. We didn't talk about guns and fighting. Not surprisingly we talked about animals, his father's old practice and the exploits of its present principal.

There was an equestrian event at Badminton that weekend. Julian was obviously eager to go, and asked if we would like to go with him. I thought for a second and replied, 'Really love to, Julian, but I'm on duty'. I wish I had a pound for every time I have made that statement in my veterinary career. I glanced at Angela, anticipating the mutual disappointment. 'Mm, well, I'm not on duty', she quipped nonchalantly. Someone said, 'Well, that's marvellous', or words to that effect, 'Saturday it is then.' Saturday came, cows went down with milk fever, and I stood them up.

We battled on in Crudwell, and at times we wondered if Hubert Evans was on our side. His was a lovely practice in a beautiful part of the country, but we could see no professional future there. Who knows, if things had been different we might still be there today. We had been part of the practice for two years, and I had gained a great deal of experience in large animal practice in a short space of time. On more than one occasion I had heard the clients' friendly comment, 'It is a two-man practice but it's run by the assistant', and I began to believe it the longer I was there.

All too often the morning plan of action began with Taff being occupied with the husbandry of his own animals. It was unusual for any livestock owner to have yards of pigs and sheep running together, but perhaps he was before his time. The yard in question was part of the Ridgeway Hospital complex that was clearly visible from our house. The shouting and bawling by a red-faced Taff as he and Sheila tried to separate lambs and pigs was an unforgettable sight. It was watched in amazement one time by my mother-in-law, who was a nurse.

'One of these days that man will drop down dead', she commented. It was not meant as a frivolous remark.

Hugh Evans had provided something in our lives which was indefinable really. He had certainly brought out the best and worst in me. I cringe now when I think back on our last disagreement. I suppose you could say that we left as we had started, rowing over pay, or to be more precise, lack of it. He had been so busy he hadn't had time to sort out my tax, well that was his excuse anyway. Adding insult to injury he had yelled, 'I cannot understand you people. Why can't you get an overdraft like me?'

Some may say he was a larger-than-life character. He certainly provided, if inadvertently, a rich number of funny stories. He was a man with vision and he knew what he wanted to achieve. In some form or other, he had built his veterinary hospital, complete with hanging baskets. He could be seen most days tending them. From our kitchen window one morning, Angela glanced out to watch him hoeing the weeds that thrived on the hospital's gravel yard. He stopped occasionally to wipe the sweat from his brow. He was working earnestly, oblivious to the fact that he was now labouring beneath a hanging basket. As he stood up he headed the prized basket like a footballer.

His face turned redder, the air turned bluer, and not surprisingly the hoe disappeared over the horizon.

CHAPTER FOUR

'TAKE ME HOME COUNTRY ROADS' – VIA CHELTENHAM SPA

Cheltenham is fashionably known as the centre of the Cotswolds. Historically it has conjured up the image and the world of the retired Army Colonel in his bath chair and its healthy spa waters. Perhaps it was once like that.

Cheltenham was not our home town, but it was our close fashionable neighbour and we had many happy memories as teenagers of letting our hair down there. The girls certainly could but it was difficult for the boys with their crew cuts. These were flat-top haircuts that impressed the girls and bemused their parents. Returning to Cheltenham in the late 1960s it was easy to recall our teenage days there in the '50s; the weekends of sunshine and swimming in the spacious outdoor lido, buying lemonade and crisps from the Art Deco buildings, and feasting as best we knew on the emerald green lawns that had been cut almost as immaculately as our hair.

The town was famous for its spa waters but the water we knew was always blue, chilly and healthy, which encouraged you to keep moving. The lido was not a place for posing. The diving boards were superb and offered you the chance to dive from the lower springboard or fixed medium boards, or, depending on your ability and how much you wanted to impress the girls, you could throw yourself off the top board in some sort of fashion. Sadly, but not surprisingly, all the diving boards have now disappeared.

Saturday nights in Cheltenham in the 1960s were terrific and we were often at the Town Hall, where local groups and sometimes the best-known rock bands in the country played. It was a rush at the end of the dance to reach St James station before the last train left for Gloucester at five minutes to midnight. The rail journey was a short one and just twenty minutes later the train pulled into Gloucester Central, where we had left our bikes with their wheels flimsily chained and secured with combination locks. Remembering any combination of numbers seemed a piece of cake back then. I am much more confident with a key nowadays.

En route the train would stop briefly at a station in a place called Churchdown, only minutes away from our destination, to let a few people off. Our eyes and noses might have been pressed harder to the steamy carriage windows if we had suspected that in just ten years or so this mysterious moonlit place would be our home for a very long time.

Our move to Cheltenham was fortuitous but was not pre-planned. We loved our years in Crudwell and were sorry to leave, but for so many reasons we knew it was time to move on. A move to any country practice would have been fine and, now a little more streetwise, we knew that knowledge of prospective employers would be more than helpful and sensible.

I scanned the job advertisements in the back pages of the *Veterinary Record* while recovering from the extraction of my tonsils at Cirencester's cottage hospital. I had been on the 'sick list' for a week following my operation. Taff eventually paid a social visit to see me at home and cheered me up by saying that he had never known anyone to take so much time off. To be honest, I had at times been forced to take to my bed for a few days on several occasions in the previous six months.

The tonsillitis I developed seemed to recur almost on a monthly cycle. It was a bit more than a nasty sore throat. My temperature soared and I quickly developed a fever that I sweated out for a day or two to the extent that Angela was removing soaking bedding and replacing them with freshly laundered sheets several times a day. The local ENT consultant had suggested an early tonsillectomy and I heartily agreed with him. My throat problem could have been resolved many months earlier had the operation taken place when it was first arranged.

'Well now, unfortunately Ivor', Taff had pontificated, 'That won't really be convenient you see.' And for some reason that I have now forgotten I was instructed to cancel the operation.

The second operation coincided with Sheila's seasonal absence. This was the time she took off from the practice to assist with haymaking on the family farm. Taff took it upon himself on that occasion to call at the hospital while he was in Cirencester and cancel the operation on my behalf. Come rain or shine I was determined there would not be a third cancellation.

The Cheltenham veterinary partnership of Hull & Eaton's advert in the back pages of the *Veterinary Record* caught my eye. As professions go, ours is a small one, and names and reputations travel quickly along the vet grapevine. Their practice premises were based in St George's Terrace, an older part of Cheltenham that we were unfamiliar with. The professional reputation of the practice was well known. In fact it was very well known, and one that a cavalier young vet today might say, 'It's worth a look at'. I thought so too, but once more it was a practice requesting and anticipating that the successful applicant would have a lot of experience tucked under his belt. I forwarded my CV but I felt it would not be prudent to enlarge too much on the experiences of my first two years in practice. I received a courteous reply to my application and an invitation for an interview from vet Tim Eaton, who at that time was the junior partner in the practice.

It was a warm August evening when we drove into Cheltenham. The sun was setting and we could not resist a drive along the famous tree-clad Promenade before our veterinary meeting. We parked near Tim's elegant home and rang the bell of his Montpellier Terrace residence. He opened the heavy decorative door and stretched out his hand. It was a firm but gentler first-meeting-handshake compared to the Crudwell introductory grasp. We sat in the luxurious lounge of Tim's house and chatted over a crystal glass of sherry, which seemed to be obligatory on these occasions, before we left for a tour of the practice premises.

Everything I had observed so far, from his shiny brown leather shoes to his immaculate brown leather briefcase, reflected efficiency and affluence. I could not help noticing with envy his brown hide medical bag sitting on the rear leather seats of his car. We followed Tim's sporty blue Alfa Romeo to his surgery premises in St George's Terrace and entered the surgery through a small green-painted door, dwarfed by the large surrounding wooden green boards, which opened on to a large cobbled yard.

At one end on the right-hand side was the practice office, a small room that was mainly taken up by a large oak table. That was clearly where the senior partner sat. Tucked away at one end behind a long black curtain was a little closet, 'for making coffee', Tim explained. He could have added that it was also the busiest room in the building. The ancient water closet was also a small room on the right off the cobbled yard. This was the second busiest room in the house. We next visited Tim's consulting room, which doubled as the operating theatre. By today's standard it was primitive, but it was also practical, clean and hygienic, and bore all the hallmarks of efficiency. I felt that I could enjoy working here.

The icing on the cake was the presence of a gaseous anaesthetic machine, something every vet takes for granted today, but at that time was like manna from heaven. This allowed operations to be carried out with the patient fast asleep in a controlled manner. Creaking rickety old stairs led from the room to a first-floor area that had once probably been a hayloft. The practice pharmacy was here and there seemed to be a drug available to treat any animal illness that you were ever likely to come across. Back on the cobbled ground floor a sliding door led to a second consulting room, an X-ray machine and a darkroom. Hull & Eaton appeared to have all the essentials that any vet could wish for. The very old buildings had the sort of appeal that perhaps today could be opened up as a veterinary museum, but at this time in history the old premises were being put to excellent use for animal welfare.

I wanted this job and couldn't wait to get started. All I needed now was the offer. I was shortly to meet the real boss and we were just a few minutes drive from his house in Charlton Kings. Like me, Peter Hull had qualified at Liverpool Vet School, and had spent nearly all of his professional life working in the Cheltenham practice. He had started his career working as a young assistant for veterinary surgeon Mr Brain in these same premises in 1945, shortly after the end of the Second World War. Peter's expertise, in keeping with most of his contemporaries, mainly revolved around farm animal medicine and the treatment of horses. I knew that he was a very experienced equine vet and an interview with him seemed daunting, as my practical work with horses, and just as importantly their owners, had been rather limited. Any fears that I might have had were unnecessary and his warm manner quickly put me at ease.

Naturally he wanted to know what I had been doing since I qualified, and the extent of my experience with farm animals and horses. I could have told him that I had stuffed four years' worth of experience into the previous two, but thought it might have sounded arrogant and would not have impressed him. So instead I related accounts of some successful cases of equine colic and lameness that I had attended and began to describe a recent and ongoing case of a lame two-year-old thoroughbred in which I was involved. Following an untimely stumble, this filly had received a deep wound to a knee and as a result of inadequate treatment by well-meaning attendants; a large granulomatous lump had developed at the wound site. For the last couple of weeks I had seen the horse at regular intervals to cauterise the lesion and to re-dress the leg. I was more than pleased with her progress.

Mr Hull looked as though he was struggling not to look too bored by my account. I had quickly suspected that we shared a similar taste in humour and undoubtedly he would have been more interested in the blarney of the Irish jockeys who assisted me in this case. I was itching to tell him that during one of the re-dressing sessions we had all downed tools to admire an attractive lady riding by on her way back from hunting. One of the Irish lads had called to her in a polite but jocular manner, 'Yer haws 'as got a real sweat on there, Madam, do you think the vet should take a look at him?'

'Don't worry, young man, it's nothing to worry about', the lady replied, 'if you had been between my legs for the last three hours you would be sweating too!'

I resisted the temptation. Messrs Hull & Eaton offered me the job, and very soon Angela and I said goodbye to Crudwell.

The three of us were on the road again. Yes, three: the third member of our family was Ginny. The stork had not visited us yet and Ginny was the beautiful yellow Labrador that we had bought from a local breeder. She was one of a litter of seven where the black labrador mum was owned by a local solicitor. He had done his homework well and chosen for their pet's mate a multi-award-winning champion dog owned by a breeder from Stow-on-the-Wold, known to most people in the dog world as

Labrador Lee. Our legal breeder's home was next door to the Wild Duck at Ewen, a well-known pub/restaurant a few miles from Cirencester.

We went along to their cottage one sunny Sunday morning when the litter was about three weeks old. The breeder escorted us to the outside kennels and called to the lovely black mum who leaped around the garden before jumping over to us. Dogs and smart Sunday clothes really do not go together. The litter of black and yellow pups seemed to leap everywhere and over each other too in their enclosed run. We spotted an inquisitive yellow female pup that seemed to take a special interest in us. Within minutes and after a vet check-up, of course, by mutual agreement we said, 'That's the one for us.' A month later pup Ginny was running around our Crudwell home and would be a very important member of our family for nearly sixteen years.

Before taking up the post in Cheltenham, letters of terms and conditions had been exchanged, and surprisingly some things had changed since our first meeting. The partners had decided to take on two new vet assistants and they were pleased to tell me that the other assistant would be Wynn Walters. By good fortune he was one of my pals from Liverpool Vet School. Things were getting better by the day, for the vet assistants anyway.

To add to his workload Mr Hull had been appointed Secretary of the British Veterinary Association, a role which inevitably meant that he would be spending much time away from his Cheltenham practice, mainly in London. To get him there in the shortest possible time he had bought a green Volvo sports car, the type some readers may still associate with The Saint, the hero of the successful 1960s detective television series of the same name. The first time I saw his car pull into the practice yard I half-expected Roger Moore to get out.

The practice had found for us a comfortable house on a relatively new estate, not far from the famous Prestbury Park racecourse of Cheltenham Gold Cup fame. Not surprisingly, Mr Hull headed the group of veterinary surgeons responsible for the welfare of the horses on race days. I was also provided with another Ford Cortina, which was one of the most popular and reliable cars on the road at the time. It was now September 1968, and I was raring to go.

My first morning's impressions in my new practice made me realise that this was how progressive vets should be doing things. I enjoyed my morning surgery, enjoyed my cup of morning coffee and looked forward to my first session of operating under modern conditions. Now there would be trained nurses to assist the surgeon. In fact they seemed to be there in abundance. Whilst preparing for my first cat spay operation, engulfed by aspiring nurses, Tim had popped his head into the operating theatre and remarked, 'Everything going OK, Ivor?' Before I could answer, he then asked, 'But do you really need the whole bloody harem to help you?' Two nurses shot off like bats out of hell. I was a little perturbed by the remark but shrugged it off quickly. There were more important things to get on with. It was the first time I had experienced his unusual sense of humour.

The silent answer to his question really was 'No, I didn't.' I just needed one good one and preferably Nikki. This bright young nurse was in many ways ahead of her time. She was a RANA (Registered Animal Nursing Auxiliary) and the first one I had worked with since I had left my Vet School. Spelt out, the title perhaps was a little demeaning and did not reflect much to anyone really, particularly to the owners of the animals, the extent of her training, nursing skills and abilities.

Eventually the veterinary profession relented to the nurses' profession's request for a more prestigious name and now they are all known as Veterinary Nurses or VNs. But the vets knew precisely who the girls in the green uniforms were, and they were highly valued members of the practice team. The vet surgeon could entrust the anaesthesia of the animal to her, and only if she were concerned would she interrupt the surgical proceedings. Oddly, there was a special cause for me to impress this RANA: Nikki's dad had been my geography master and a Crypt School athletic coach. It's a small world!

Most Monday and Thursday mornings I would be found in my farm gear carrying out the annual tuberculin test on a herd of cattle somewhere within a 20-mile radius of Cheltenham. The routine was to check over the health of every animal in the herd, measure the thickness of the skin in the neck region and give two injections under the skin. Three day later you returned to the farm, a second inspection was carried out and any reactions at the injection sites were recorded, and in this way, depending on the degree of skin swelling, any cattle infected with TB could be identified. It was a tedious task and was, at that time, most unusual to find an animal that even suggested it had been in contact with the disease.

How things have changed. Forty years later there is a very high risk of animals in the herd being infected. The numbers of cattle affected have grown beyond imagination and the reason for this is now an ongoing argument among farmers, vets, DEFRA (Department for Environment, Food and Rural Affairs), and wildlife conservationist groups speaking on behalf of the badger, which in one way or another is involved in the spread of the disease. The cattle testing continued on Tuesdays and Fridays; those were Wynn's testing days. I particularly looked forward to these days, knowing I would spend most of my time in the operating theatre. But not before we had enjoyed the end of morning surgery coffee break.

The location of the surgery premises had an additional bonus; it was opposite Cheltenham's long-established Locke's Bakery and you arrived at work each morning to the wonderful aroma of freshly baked bread. Before 10 o'clock a nurse had taken the staff's orders and returned to the surgery with a large bag of hot doughnuts oozing raspberry jam. It was an enjoyable start to the day. A cup of strong coffee and two doughnuts later it was time to begin the operating session. Back then, I could eat as many doughnuts I wanted back then and it seemed to make no difference at all to the old waistline. Today I daren't eat any.

The operations invariably started with the neutering of cats. Cat castrations were quick and simple and that is why they were normally first on the list. Next came their female counterparts: cat spays were usually second on the list. Strangely this daily routine is the one I would still practise today. Perhaps it is the surgeon's way of warming up. Dog castrations followed and finally the bitch spays. In the hands of a competent surgeon, this operation can justifiably be described as a routine procedure. It is nevertheless one of the most demanding operations that any vet is likely to carry out and the opportunities for surgical disaster are numerous – not to mention the all-important safe administration of a general anaesthetic for half an hour or so.

My mind frequently drifted back to the Crudwell operating theatre and Sheila steadfastly holding a young bitch patient about to receive her intravenous barbiturate injection that would induce general anaesthesia long enough to carry out a routine hysterectomy. There the anaesthetic of choice (in truth the only one available to me) was Nembutal – pentobarbitone sodium. It was recognised as being a reliable and 'reasonably safe' anaesthetic, whatever that meant. It was not recommended for use in aged animals but nobody ever seemed to know how old 'aged' was. My college notes reminded me that the dose was $\frac{1}{5}$ grain per pound body weight, and that applied to healthy animals between 25lb and 35lb. In animals below 25lb the dose needed to be slightly decreased, and in animals above 35lb, slightly increased. Sometimes calculating the dose seemed to take as long as the operation itself, and at the start of every operating session I prayed that Taff's scales and my maths were reasonably accurate. The hand-held calculator had yet to be invented. My confidence was boosted by experiencing only minor surgical and post-operative calamities, but it was not that unusual for an owner to ring up the next day asking if their drowsy, staggering pet should now have come round from the anaesthetic.

The Cheltenham experience was a little different to my Crudwell days. The nurse passed a syringe filled with a pre-calculated dose of a short-acting barbiturate and the sedated patient fell asleep rapidly as I gave the intravenous injection of thiopentone. I popped an endotracheal tube through the open larynx, connected up to the anaesthetic machine supplying a regulated amount of halothane gas, and, hey presto, we had an anaesthetic utopia, and it was all systems go. I enjoyed surgery and Tim obligingly gave me a free hand in what I did. The operations were numerous and varied and on most days there was a reasonable justification to delve into a cat or dog's abdomen.

I am sure that almost every day one of the vets in the practice would remove a small rubber ball from a dog's stomach or a chop bone that had reached the small intestine. The X-ray images, as you can imagine, were spectacular and we regularly returned to the owner an object retrieved from the digestive tract that had been missing for days or even weeks. Occasionally an owner would be totally adamant that they had no idea how their pet came across the foreign body in the first place. Top of the list in this department was the condom, which most vets will have removed from a dog's digestive system at some time in their career. It's amazing where the dogs find them. Fortunately pet owners today are much more aware of what their pet can safely eat and play with.

Gastric and intestinal foreign bodies are scarcer in cats, mainly due to their more fastidious eating habits. One of the more common objects removed from the cat's digestive system was the sewing needle.

Kittens love to play with cotton but do not know how to deal with the sharp thing attached at one end.

Cheltenham's animals seemed to have at least their fair share of road traffic accidents (RTAs) and as a result almost every day we faced another distraught owner across the examination table. Our practice was as well equipped as most of the day to tackle these problems. Orthopaedic cases became a challenge and putting broken limbs back together by pinning and plating fractured bones, and removing damaged hips, was almost a daily routine. Every basic bone operation stimulated the desire and the challenge to do the next more demanding task. There is just one way to gain experience.

Not all bone fractures required orthopaedic surgery and there were numerous occasions when applying a Plaster of Paris cast under a general anaesthetic was adequate to immobilise a limb long enough to allow a minor fracture to heal satisfactorily. This was the case one day when I had applied a plaster cast to a young Boxer dog that had received a bump in a minor road accident. I discussed the treatment with the owner, who lived in the St Paul's area of Cheltenham, and gave the appropriate post-op instructions, followed by the usual afterthought, 'If you are worried at all about anything, give us a ring.'

When the telephone rang at 11 o'clock that night the last thing I imagined I would hear was, 'For Christ's sake get here quick mister, he's grown another bleedin' leg!' I was about to say 'Pull the other one', when I recognised the genuine panic in the caller's voice. I parked up under a bright streetlamp and walked down the road to the owner, who was leaning on his wooden gate puffing away ferociously on a cigarette.

'He was all right earlier, but when we went into the kitchen later on he had five legs!'

It was difficult to keep a straight face. I examined my lively patient on the kitchen floor. I do not know how, but he had somehow managed to remove his injured leg from the plaster cast. With the original leg shape of the cast intact and still attached firmly to his shoulder and chest, the illusion was perfect. I explained to the owners, who were now recovering from their shock, that it would be necessary to apply another cast and agreed to keep him sedated for a couple of days until he was used to the cast. I wished them goodnight as the reassured owner lit up another cigarette.

There was one particular RTA to which I have to confess guilt and embarrassment. Towards the end of a busy day I had called in for a quick afternoon cup of tea with Angela at our home, a semi-detached house on the Wyman's Brook estate. I drove off to evening surgery along Swindon Lane and was astonished by a black cat that appeared from nowhere and was determined to get across the road before I arrived at his starting point. The cat lost the race and I felt a bump on my nearside. I jumped out of my car – thinking that at least he can't complain about the veterinary service – with the intention of whizzing rapidly back to surgery with my patient, but he had disappeared. I spent the next twenty minutes searching for him without success.

'I've done my best old chap, wherever you may be', I muttered to myself, hoping that he hadn't gone to the great cats' resting place in the sky.

However, to my great relief he was still very much in this world and an hour later an extremely worried lady from Swindon Lane presented her rather subdued and wobbly black cat in my surgery, complete with a prominent bump on his head. He was a little concussed but was suffering from nothing worse than that and I knew he would make a complete recovery.

'Do you think he's been in a car accident, Mr Smith?' his owner asked?

'Yes I do, Mrs Jones, there's no doubt about that', I replied, as I gave the cat an antibiotic and painkilling injection, 'but I don't think he's too badly hurt and I am sure he will be back to normal in a couple of days.'

My sympathetic comments were not enough to prevent her angry rhetoric on car owners who drive too fast and hadn't the decency to stop after hitting a poor animal. I agreed wholeheartedly, but in fact I hadn't been driving that fast and her cat did seem hellbent on destruction, and I did stop afterwards. How could I possibly give her a bill knowing that I was responsible for the accident? I don't know, but I did, and it's played heavily on my conscience for the last forty years, occasionally.

Wynn and I settled quickly into the routine of being the practice assistants. During the week we were each on duty for two nights and alternated the Friday and weekend duties. One of the partners acted as back-up for those rare occasions in the middle of the night when clients needed you to be in two places at the same time. One morning in the very early hours Wynn hauled himself out of bed to attend a cow having a difficult time calving. He called at the surgery en route to the farm to collect instruments and the ropes and tackle he needed to do the job. Most of it was stored in one of the upstairs rooms at the top of the creaky wooden staircase. He had been sorting out gear for about ten minutes when he was more than a little perturbed to hear heavy breathing and footsteps creeping up the stairs. Feeling a little perturbed was not quite how he described his anxiety to me, instead he thought he was sitting on bricks and his intestinal spasms only stopped when he discovered that it wasn't the surgery phantom coming up the stairs but Mr Hull. He too was relieved to find his assistant upstairs and not a couple of burglars. He had come for some calving gear because, against the odds, two farmers had telephoned within minutes of each other at 2.30 a.m., both wanting the vet out to calve a cow. Most night-time visits to farms involved the inevitable problems that went hand-in-hand with farming; the difficult calvings, the milk fevers and other metabolic diseases associated with the high milk-producing cow, and which were normal events even on the best of dairy farms. Sometimes there was an evening visit to cases that were truly avoidable.

One such occasion was a visit to see a group of young Friesian steers that had been castrated a week or so before. The operation, if you can call it that, had been carried out by the owner using an instrument called an emasculator. The technique, carried out legally by a skilled operator, results in relatively little discomfort to the young animal and within hours the calf's behaviour returns to normal. The pinching of the skin surrounding the structures that lead to the testicles in the jaws of the instrument causes the speedy disappearance of the animal's masculinity. It is a simple and safe way of castrating young calves. It was never meant to be used as a method of castrating cattle approaching maturity, but this is exactly what had been attempted on this occasion.

I arrived at a small field enclosure near Andoversford at about 7.30 on a warm summer's evening where I had arranged to meet the farmer. I was not prepared for what greeted me. Two of the ten young bulls were already dying and it was clear that a couple more, even with treatment, would soon join them. It would at least be relief from the agony they were suffering. The testicles of each of the animals were swollen to at least four times their normal size. Some seemed to resemble little footballs and serum and blood-tinged pus oozed from the traumatised skin where an attempt had been made to sever the spermatic cords a week or so ago. Flies buzzed around the wounds in the evening sun. The animals seemed past caring and most showed some of the classic signs of bovine tetanus. The toxins produced by the clostridial tetanus bacteria were causing acute muscular spasms and a rigidity that caused the wretched animals to feel as though they walked on stilts. Others were recumbent, bloated and cruelly dying unnecessarily of tetanus.

I arranged for several of the cattle to be shot and within hours their misery and suffering ended. The remainder I loaded to the maximum with antibiotics, analgesics, tetanus anti-serum and anything else I had in the boot I thought might be helpful. I hoped the farmer would still be paying off his vet's bill five years later.

Although this kind of farming atrocity was fortunately a rarity, there were others of the same ilk who somehow or other always seemed to find some way of avoiding prosecution. That said, however, I enjoyed the farm side of the practice enormously.

Young vets thought a lot about their cars back then and undoubtedly do today. How you reached a particular farm or how quickly you attended an emergency situation was important. Wynn sensibly drove his own reliable Hillman Minx and the practice funded the running costs. I had opted to drive the practice's Ford Cortina even though I knew it had a chequered history. We knew the previous driver. He was a very likeable assistant vet named Mike Hinton, who was leaving the practice to take up a position with MAFF (Ministry of Agriculture, Fisheries and Food), the government department known today as DEFRA. For some inexplicable reason Mike didn't get on too well with this car and it seemed to spend more time off the road than on it. On one occasion the gears failed, or at least some part of the system did, and Mr Hull was surprised when his assistant walked into his office with a Cortina gearstick in his hand. Once Mike had the misfortune to be involved in an accident that resulted in considerable damage to the front end of the car. The practice philosophically repaired the damage and soon he was off again in the car to do his farm rounds.

Soon after the last event Mike was carrying out a cattle TB herd test on a local farm near Charlton Kings and had parked on the steep Ham Hill. In the middle of the morning the driverless Cortina decided to roll boot-first down the hill and Mike and the farmer could only watch in amazement as the car picked up speed. Eventually it came to a stop against a collapsing brick wall. This time it was just the *rear* end of the car that needed replacing. It was believed that the handbrake had failed.

The practice back-up vehicle was a super white Austin Mini. Driving this little car was tremendous fun and most members of staff found regular excuses to go out in it. One afternoon when the Cortina was off the road again, on this occasion for a routine service, I jumped into the Mini and headed out of Cheltenham through Battledown towards Hewletts Farm, and was soon climbing Harp Hill and Aggs Hill. As I rounded one corner I was a bit surprised to see a Morris Minor descending the hill towards me, on the same side of the road. It wasn't quite *déjà vu* Crudwell, despite the screech of brakes, but there was the now-familiar sound of bending metal and breaking glass. I stepped out of the Mini to confront the hysterical lady driver. She got in first.

'Oh my God', she wailed. 'What on earth will my husband say?' There was only one thing I could think of.

'What does your husband usually say to you when you drive on the wrong side of the road?' Back at her house and after half an hour of telephone calls to the six most important people in her world whilst swigging a large G&T, I finally had the chance to ring my practice office. Later, I eventually arrived at Hewletts Farm and offered the farmer a strange excuse for being an hour late to disbud and castrate his calves. The young cattle no doubt appreciated the delay and enjoyed their last hour of uninterrupted manhood.

Most days passed quickly and were happily rewarding. I would often arrive home to be told by Angela; 'Have a quick shower because we're meeting up with Tom, Dick, Harry and Wynn and the wives for a bite to eat at 8 at the usual place.' Eating out was starting to become part and parcel of our social life in Cheltenham. The 'usual place' could well have been one of several popular local pub steak houses. It was probably the start of the cafeteria society and the adventurous type of restaurateur that remains popular today, and none could be more so than the young couple who ran Bistro 42. Unsurprisingly, this immensely popular eating house could be found at no. 42 on the High Street.

Bistro food was a little different from the usual restaurant menus of the time. The meals were generally meaty, spicy, and invariably cooked in French wine. We were happy to eat by flickering candlelight, sitting on old benches and stools at bare wooden tables. Glass ashtrays were naturally in abundance. The walls were decorated with numerous modern art prints to stimulate chat in case you ran out of conversation, interspersed with solid metallic items, including heavy brass circular objects resembling medieval shields.

One memorable evening found Wynn and me with our young wives and some friends sitting under one of the bistro's prize bronzes putting the farming and veterinary world to rights. At a convenient time Wynn and I excused ourselves to take a trip to the gents' and at that very moment the enormous brass ornament above us inexplicably decided to part company with its wall fixture. It must have been one of the most fortuitous calls of nature ever. Broken glasses, ashtrays, cutlery and china flew in all directions as the enormous shield smashed down onto the space we had just vacated.

Later that same evening the appetites of some of the diners in the restaurant were tested to the limit. I was pleasantly surprised to discover that I had met our young waitress earlier in the day. I'd had the pleasure of castrating her beloved cat at the surgery that morning.

'Oh, you're Ivor Smith, aren't you?' our waitress exclaimed. I nodded acknowledgement.

'You operated on Hendrix today, didn't you?' she announced loudly to everyone in the restaurant.

'I certainly did', I replied. 'How is he this evening?'

'Oh he's fine now I'm sure, but he disgraced himself when we got him home. His tummy was really upset,' she said a little more quietly.

'Nothing to worry about really', I told her reassuringly. 'Vomiting is often a problem after a general anaesthetic.'

'Oh no, he wasn't sick', she corrected, speaking more loudly now. 'It was the other end; there was stinky diarrhoea everywhere! It was me being sick!'

I cringed and hoped that no one in the restaurant had been put off their mulligatawny soup.

Regrettably, this inappropriate restaurant banter was just one of the first of its kind for me, and many more appetite-ending conversations would take place over the years. Restaurants are fine places to bump into clients and have a social chat but, before saying hello, I soon learned to rack my brains to be sure I remembered their pets' ailments and hoped that above everything else, digesting their food satisfactorily was not a problem.

The 1960s social life in Cheltenham was fantastic. When Ange and I were not eating we were partying. Deep down we knew these halcyon days were numbered and it was a time of packing in the fun while we still could. An immensely popular annual event at the Town Hall was the Students' Arts Ball. Naturally it was a fancy dress event, and one memorable year the theme was the Time of the Romans. Unsurprisingly, most revellers dressed in the style of the corrupt and debauched era of the Fall of the Roman Empire. Our band of centurions, gladiators and slave girls met for a warm-up drink in a subterranean bar at a well-known Irish pub on Montpellier. An hour or so later, the fortified slave women led the way towards the direction of the Town Hall and the ball. The skirted centurions and Roman riff-raff followed. Lagging behind I stopped halfway up the stairs to to the Town Hall to tie a flapping bootlace. As I was bending down, a centurion climbing the stairs behind me passed by and, looking back, uttered with relief, 'Oh, thank God for that, it's a bloke. For a moment I thought it was the hairiest woman's legs I'd ever seen in my life!'

The ball ended in the early hours and soup was served at about 4 a.m. For most it was sobering sustenance for the journey home. For one of us it was breakfast before the equally sobering telephone rang again, probably in less than two hours' time. Soon we would be back with the animals.

Each day we routinely dealt with the problems of pets, farm animals and loveable ponies, and on the whole we felt that our efforts were truly appreciated. Yet some of the horse-owning fraternity were a breed of their own. There was a type of owner who seemed to have more money than sense, was ridiculously demanding and believed they had more knowledge of horse medicine than any vet on the planet. Certainly heaps more than one particular vet whom had only been qualified a few years.

One occasion that springs to mind arose on a Friday afternoon when Mr Hull was returning from his BVA secretarial duties in London. When I returned to the surgery after lunch Tim grabbed me and said almost apologetically that Mrs Fitzroy-something or other wanted a visit without delay to look at a hunter that had now been lame for a couple of days. It was a forty-five minute drive to her Cotswold residence some 20 miles beyond bustling Cirencester, and a further couple of minutes up the drive to the magnificent historic house. I eventually pulled into the stable yard and it became immediately obvious from her aloof presence whose horse I had come to see. I opened my car door as she approached and prepared to introduce myself, as we hadn't met before. She was clearly expecting Peter Hull. It took all of five seconds to realise that I was not welcome.

'Who are you?' she demanded, in a way that suggested that the plum in her mouth was the largest ever grown. I suspected she knew darn well who I was without further explanation.

'Well, I am Mr Hull's veterinary assistant and I have come to . . .'

'Nobody other than Mr Hull looks at my horses', she interrupted, 'so don't bother to get out of your car.'

I could easily have said the pleasure was all mine as I turned round and headed back to Cheltenham. I was cross and frustrated by the woman's arrogance. No doubt Mr Hull would attend in person at the earliest opportunity, but in the meantime the lame horse would remain in discomfort, possibly developing an increasingly severe infection. Who knows?

Despite having to tolerate a few difficult horse owners, the majority were fun characters and enjoyable to work with. One in particular was a wealthy businessman farmer who had moved to the Boddington area from the Midlands and spoke with a strong regional accent. At times he could be a bit of a tartar but I got on well with him and his large family. The farm was mainly a dairy one, but it was clear that his main interest was his racehorses. One day I was asked to examine a horse called Ward Arms that was becoming increasingly sluggish in training. A clinical examination revealed nothing of significance and the usual action under these circumstances was to give the traditional symptomatic treatment, an injection of vitamin B12. It did no harm and often seemed to do some good.

Perhaps to demonstrate I was a little enterprising I thought I would give the horse something extra, this being a big oily shot of anabolic steroids which were just becoming available. Today it is illegal to administer these to improve performance but it was quite permissible at the time and I gave the biggest dose that I could within the limits of the pharmaceutical company's recommended doses. Ward Arms ran at the end of that week. I cannot remember what the odds against him were, but he won by a mile. I was quite popular on that farm for a long time.

We took our work seriously and as professionally as young vets could, but from time to time things happened that our governing body would have frowned upon. Ignorance was not bliss as far as the Royal College of Veterinary Surgeons was concerned. How they may have reacted to a complaint about me driving to Cheltenham with a body part hanging from the back of my car we shall fortunately never know.

Christine was a good trainee nurse in the practice who understood the needs of the animals and their owners. She also had a wicked sense of humour. One particular client of the practice enjoyed eating calf's sweetmeats and when the occasion arose Christine was able to provide him with the main ingredients for his supper. For those who are neither gourmets nor French, sweetmeats are calves' testicles.

I had spent one bright, crisp spring morning at Stockwell Farm, a large dairy farm near Birdlip, and on this occasion was ably assisted by the farm's stockmen and Christine. We had gradually carried out castration of a large group of calves using a technique known as the open method. Without going into unnecessary detail the method entailed removing the essential organs completely. At the end of the morning we had operated on about a hundred calves and naturally ended up with twice that number of testicles. They had been placed temporarily into a bucket and as we prepared to leave the farm I could see that considerate Christine had the appetite of our carnivorous client in mind.

'He's in for a bit more than a beanfeast here', I muttered to myself. Clearly she wanted to offer these delicacies to the client in some more appetising way than in a bucket – not that that was particularly important I am sure, providing they were fresh. She delved into the boot and found a pink plastic arm-length glove of the type normally worn to protect the vet's arm when carrying out a manual internal examination of a cow. One by one each little testicle was delicately transferred from the bucket to the glove and the first lot slid into the plastic fingers. Gradually, as more were added, the pulpy hand took shape and the glove began to take on the appearance of a severed arm. Our job done, we bid farewell to the chaps on the farm. Christine had obligingly put all the equipment, overalls, wellies and bloody, testicle-filled glove into the boot of the car and off we journeyed back to base, no doubt accompanied by the Rolling Stones on the radio.

Half an hour later we pulled into the practice yard, both of us ready for lunch. Going round to the boot to unload our equipment, I not only lost my appetite but my thoughts turned to the cars parked behind us as we halted at numerous traffic lights on the A46. I could not believe that we had driven all the way back with the glove dangling from the boot, looking for all the world like a gory human arm.

CHAPTER FIVE

PIONEER SETTLERS

I know that this is a strange chapter title for a book on veterinary life, but all will soon be revealed. Actually, the circumstances prompting these words won't be revealed until the last chapter, but by then I hope that you have not become so thoroughly bored with my story that you won't read that far.

The drive to work each morning entailed a fast route through St Paul's, passing the old Cheltenham maternity hospital and the lower High Street; it was the shortest route to St George's Terrace, the freshly baked bread and jam-oozing doughnuts, and the veterinary surgery of Hull & Eaton.

There was an optional journey through the town which took you along the famous Promenade. It took a little longer and at about 8.30 in the morning was particularly hazardous, especially for young male drivers who for some reason became oblivious to the vehicle in front. It was the time of day when Cheltenham's young women were also on their way to work. It was also that time in history when the miniskirt was in vogue. The epidemic of minor motor accidents in that area that resulted from admiring glances was so rife that the insurance claims departments began to refer to them as the Promenade mini-shunt.

Cheltenham life was fun, and as carefree youngsters Angela and I enjoyed it while we could, although we were always aware that before too long we would have the trappings of mortgages, parenthood and the responsibility of running our own practice, but at this stage we had no real idea where that practice might be. Life began to move in a different and more serious direction the day Wynn handed in his notice. It was now our third year in the practice and both Wynn and I suspected that, frustratingly, we would not be offered partnerships in the foreseeable future. Whenever the subject was raised the topic of conversation was quickly changed. We had worked hard and were aware of just how much the practice had grown in the time that we had been there. We were ambitious and knew that for both of us our veterinary world was about to change dramatically.

Wynn made the first move and became a junior partner in a successful practice in Chippenham. To make matters worse for me, his departure coincided with the end of Mr Hull's BVA full-time commitments and his return to the practice sadly seemed to justify the decision not to find a replacement for Wynn. My working hours increased rapidly and the situation was aggravated by Tim Eaton becoming heavily involved in the British Small Animal Veterinary Association. The partners' prestigious positions in these paramount organisations were tremendous kudos for the practice but the grass-roots work still had to be done. For a while I felt privileged to have their trust and enjoyed the responsibility of running their practice virtually single-handed for several days at a time. But no matter how much you enjoy your work there is a limit as to how much you can do without a rest and some sleep.

Eventually I had to admit defeat. At 8 o'clock one Monday morning I drove into the practice's cobbled yard, leaned back as far as I could in my car seat and dozed off, waiting for Peter's return from his London job. I hadn't slept for more than a couple of hours in one go since Thursday night. That was three days ago! The telephone had not stopped ringing all weekend. Eventually I felt that every cow on every farm had a difficult calving and if she didn't she would just go down with milk fever anyway, just to keep me awake and on my toes. It wasn't quite as bad as that, but it was taxing enough to drain every ounce of my energy reserves.

I knew that Mr Hull was due back by 9 o'clock and I eagerly awaited his return, but dreaded having to explain to him how I felt and that I just couldn't carry on without some rest. It sounded wimpish, but my case was probably supported by my drained white face and lips that had started to break out in numerous painful ulcers. The green Volvo sports car finally drew up and I was relieved to see Peter emerging. He saw straight away that I wasn't fit to carry on and simply told me to go home and come back when I was up to it again.

I was worried enough to make an appointment to see a doctor that day. My own doctor was on holiday and I was examined by his brash young locum. Actually I wasn't examined at all. I might have felt more reassured if he had at least stuck a thermometer in my mouth. After two minutes of irrelevant questions his diagnosis was that I had a viral infection. I suggested to him that, before I dropped down dead, perhaps it would be in order for me to have a few days at home.

'No, you'll be far better off at work than lounging around at home', the doctor announced unsympathetically.

With my final ounce of strength I managed to convince him that I was truly knackered and with or without his blessing I was not going back to work, so he signed me off for a week. I spent most of that week sleeping, and when I wasn't sleeping I was thinking really hard about the future.

I returned to work refreshed a week later and was quickly back in the swing of things once more. It was an unusual week, as things turned out. Churchdown is about 6 miles from Cheltenham, a small ancient village tucked away between Cheltenham and Gloucester. Here there were a number of family-run farms and smallholdings, some of which were run by local folk I knew. On that particular Monday morning I found myself at Green Farm in the company of the Halford family, father Albert and son John. I was there to carry out the annual herd TB test. It would take most of the morning to inspect and inject the cattle if things went well. As it turned out the task was completed by early afternoon, having moved the groups of cattle from Green Farm to other associated farms in the village, as well as some disassociated farms, gardens and allotments, repairing numerous fences on the way.

I found myself on the village green once more on the following Thursday morning, measuring the skin of cattle necks. The second day of the test is normally a shorter affair but it provided the farmer with a veterinary visit paid for by the government and thus the opportunity to get some routine work done at a bargain price. It was rare for a farmer ever to miss this opportunity. On this occasion, after the official Ministry business was completed, we dehorned some cattle. Removing the horns from adult cattle was not just fashionable at the time, but sensible; cattle without horns were less likely to bully other animals and made handling them safer. Having anaesthetised the horns of each animal they were again put into the steel cattle crush which restrained their movements and made it possible to remove the horns by sawing them off at the base with a tenon saw.

The restraint sounds ideal, but it is surprising the range of movements that a crush-restrained bovine can display. On this occasion one managed to penetrate my forehead with the pointed tip of its horn. A mixture of blood and perspiration trickled down my face. I am sure it must have looked dramatic. Job done, I returned to the surgery anticipating a sympathetic response from the nurses. I walked slowly past two of them and neither took the slightest notice of me. I would have got more attention from even the most biased of rugby referees if I'd shouted 'Did you see that, Ref?' I washed my face and went home for lunch.

I found myself back in Churchdown on several occasions that week. Between testing Mr Halford's cattle I had been sent out to White House Farm to see one of Mr Lever's lame cows and whilst there his sons John and Ken asked me if there was time for me to look at another lame cow. I obliged and from somewhere they produced several more cows which were 'not exactly lame but walking, you know, a bit different'. My planned half-hour visit turned into a 2½-hour foot-trimming session. My back aches today even just thinking about it, but the following two-hour chat was to lead to events I had previously only dreamt of. The conversation was a mixture of the usual farming doom and gloom and local gossip, but more importantly their vision of the future of Churchdown.

By the end of that week I was 100 per cent sure I knew what I wanted to do. I would start my own practice in Churchdown. I was going to be the Village Vet.

Around the time I entered Vet School, whenever I was back home in Gloucestershire, Angela and I often wandered over one of our favourite places, Chosen Hill. It was a wonderful location where you could get away from it all and plan your future, which in our case we hoped might include a veterinary utopia. Our favourite walk took us out of

Hucclecote along a winding lane towards Churchdown, past the old farmhouse of the De Lisle Wells family at Noake Court and the imposing Chosen Hill House, taking us eventually to the Bat & Ball pub.

A lemonade and half a pint of bitter later, we wandered back to Angela's Hucclecote home on the other side of Chosen Hill. We often found ourselves looking down the hill and admiring the attractive new houses in Crifty Craft Lane and beyond them the miles of green fields and endless open land. Occasionally the stillness was interrupted by the distant whistle and puff of steam from the engine of a passing steam train. On one occasion I remarked,

'Do you know, Ange, this would be a lovely place to have our own practice.' A true word is often spoken in jest, but on this occasion I think I was really serious.

These youthful romantic notions were not at the top of my thoughts as my calloused hands pared away at the feet of John and Ken's cattle, but the financial realities were. Our profession was an odd one and it had only slowly crept into the hard-headed twentieth-century business world. The idea that the treatment of animals could possibly be equated with making anything other than a living seemed outrageous to many. It was Mr Hull who first said to me, 'Ivor, you'll need to be a businessman first and a practising veterinary surgeon second, or it won't be very long before you will be a practising veterinary surgeon without a business.' The first time I heard him say that my thoughts returned to the Crudwell practice and my early chats with local farmers. Apparently it was not unusual for Mr Pettifer to send out a bill to a farm client about every three years for their perusal.

As I pared away at the overgrown feet I couldn't help wondering why there had never been a veterinary practice here in Churchdown. I returned to base later that afternoon and joined the queues of rush-hour traffic, which seemed to grow ever longer as time went by. An emergency call at this time of the day meant a frustrating twenty minutes' delay trying to get out of Cheltenham. 'Bet I wouldn't have this problem in Churchdown', I thought to myself.

One evening that week the telphone rang at about 11 o'clock, and half an hour later I was attending an emergency in Churchdown. There was nothing particularly unusual about the treatment of this case and an hour or so later I was back in Cheltenham, operatingon an elderly mongrel bitch who was struggling in vain to produce her few, but very large, puppies. When I later said goodnight to the owners, as they left with their sleepy dog and three new pups, my mind was made up. I was going to become the Churchdown vet.

Once the seeds were sown I couldn't get the idea of putting up my plate out of my head. Angela gradually got used to the idea of what might be in store and as the weeks went by her early doubts changed to cautious enthusiasm. Perhaps in hindsight, with a pregnant wife and a baby son, the timing was not perfect. But perhaps if we always wait for the perfect moment we may never do anything.

We drove to Churchdown most evenings and weekends when the opportunity arose searching for suitable premises. In our minds we knew the sort of building we were looking for. We definitely needed a roof over our heads, but essentially we needed premises that could be converted into a veterinary surgery. We had approached the planning department of Tewkesbury Borough Council but the young fellow delegated to advise us on the sort of property we should be looking for knew little about animals and nothing about their behaviour or needs. In order to minimise the social distress he perceived would be associated with a veterinary surgery (the constant barking of dogs and obnoxious odours), he directed us ever closer to the top of Chosen Hill. At times, as a safety margin, I thought he was directing us a few miles further on to neighbouring Coopers Hill and Robinswood Hill.

How we initially found The Brambles I really cannot remember now. It must have been advertised somewhere. In 1971 property across the country was rocketing in price and houses changed hands so quickly the estate agents only ever bothered to put up a 'Sold' board. I do remember telephoning the owners of an interesting turn-of-the-century Victorian house that might possibly suit our needs. The house and huge garden belonged to Major and Mrs Farlow who had lived there for the previous thirteen years. At the appointed time on a gorgeous late autumn afternoon we were greeted at the front door by Mrs Farlow, and having introduced ourselves we were immediately invited to view the second floor rooms first. We walked into one of the rear bedrooms where she had drawn the blinds to protect the furnishings from the brilliant low October sun. She dramatically drew back the curtains and we were presented with a magnificent display of the Major's gardening achievements.

In the foreground the lawns rolled back to meet the weedless vegetable garden beyond. Angela and I dared a subtle glance at each other, one of disbelief at our good fortune. Our reaction was noticed by the observant Mrs Farlow.

'The garden a little too big for you?' she enquired, in an almost maternal way.

'Oh no, not at all', I replied. 'We like gardening.' We did like gardening very much, but I must have sounded stupidly naïve. If only she had known what I wanted to do to her garden. Before leaving the bedroom, and with a private knowing wink to Angela, I assured Mrs Farlow of our total interest and, within minutes and probably to her astonishment, I boldly announced 'We'll buy it!'

We had no idea where the money would come from. We made an offer via our solicitor which was a little below the fortune we thought we were being asked for, and were delighted when it was accepted.

The estate agent dispensed with the formality of the 'For Sale' board, and simply put up the 'Sold' board that week. At the same time I arranged an appointment with the manager of a building society on Cheltenham Promenade. We went through the usual checklist and things went well until he began asking relevant questions such as, 'What will be your income?' The answer was that I might soon not have one and within a couple of months I might even be on social security.

I am grateful that the office computer wasn't yet in use, or at this point all the lights would be flashing crazily before it exploded and I was politely escorted to the front door. Fortunately at this time there was still an opportunity for a little negotiation, debate and discretion, and with a bit of persuasion we secured our mortgage. However, we still had to obtain planning consent. We arranged to visit the chairman of the Churchdown Parish Council. A room was set aside for such meetings and we took our place on a bench in the chairman's monastic consulting room in his secluded Green Lane House. He listened carefully and with interest to our proposal. We believed that we had something to offer the village and his response was incredibly positive.

With the support of the Parish Council we soon had our planning go-ahead. We sold our Cheltenham home, made a small profit which would be our sole starting capital sum, and moved to Churchdown.

We moved into The Brambles on a bright yet bitterly cold January morning in 1972. It did not take long to move the furniture in, as we hadn't got much. The house had been empty for a couple of weeks with all the windows shut and secured, which had caused a musty odour that was quickly resolved by opening the windows in every room. This was a mixed blessing as we had chosen to move in during one of the coldest winter spells for many years. We were convinced of this as, later that night, we huddled around a back room stove that provided one room with bearable warmth and the house with some hot water. We wondered if the Farlows had ever heard about gas boilers and central heating.

The next few weeks were bedlam. Tewkesbury Borough Council had approved our surgery development plans and on our first Sunday morning in Churchdown, Norman and his gang arrived. The lads were ready for a speedy brick-laying session and the walls of our first surgery were erected in five hours flat, in time for them to shoot off to their local for a lunchtime beer. Norman and his wife had been our good neighbours for a couple of years in Cheltenham. He was a skilled bricklayer, but his talents didn't extend to animal management, although he enjoyed giving a piece of sandwich to Ginny when the opportunity arose.

One summer when his wife went away for a couple of weeks, her last words to him as she left the house were, 'Don't forget to feed the budgie, Norman.' The budgie had been moved to a cool bedroom during her absence. She returned two weeks later and her first words on entering the house were 'How's Charlie, Norman?' For the first time in a fortnight Norman remembered they had a budgie called Charlie. The reality of the situation was that they *did* have a budgie called Charlie. It was another couple of weeks before Norman was sure he still had a wife.

It took just three weeks for the building to transform into a surgery. Actually, built on a shoestring budget, I thought it was really good. All the essentials were there. I proudly put my plate up on the front of the house. It was not the traditional brass plate. Instead I chose a fashionable brushed stainless steel version adorned by dark oak backing. We were perhaps a little optimistically hoping that we would be far too busy to polish it with Brasso every day. Amazingly this was the limit of our advertising our presence to the village and potential clients. Any step beyond this and I would be appearing before the Royal

College of Veterinary Surgeons' Disciplinary Committee, with more than an evens chance of being struck off the Register. Thirty-odd years down the line the situation seems almost comical but at the time it was a problem always on a vet's mind. What would I have given then for a full-page entry in the *Yellow Pages* or a jingle on the local radio?

It was the opinion of the Royal College that word of mouth and recommendation from existing clients should be the only way to achieve professional success. This is a tricky situation when you have no existing clients, but as in most villages there was plenty of word of mouth, whatever was being said. The early weeks were spent building in the surgery and in the house. Most of the work was subcontracted to skilled tradesmen, but there always seemed to be many in-between jobs for which no one claimed responsibility. My student days spent on building sites were once more put to good use.

I accept that my building experience was limited and I had never removed a fireplace before. This became clear one dreadful afternoon. My hammering and chiselling was interrupted when son Ed, who had now reached the crawling stage, managed to find a gap in the roped-off rails of the first floor landing and squeezed through. His 12-foot fall on to a stone tiled floor was, thankfully, broken by his folded pushchair. Angela rushed him directly to the doctor and I returned to my fireplace. I finally succeeded in dismantling the old thing, but at one stage I had ended up underneath it. When it started to move I had no idea how heavy a fireplace could be and the intact structure had a will of its own. Despite my best muscular efforts it settled across one of my legs. During this commotion and while I was cursing and swearing, the doorbell rang.

I hobbled to the door and a concerned elderly lady asked me if I was the owner of a Labrador dog that had just been hit by a car. By her side was an even more worried-looking Ginny. I immediately forgot my own aches and pains and while I checked her over, Angela returned from the doctor's surgery smiling. Ginny, Ed and I had all managed to escape with just a few cuts and bruises, some more painful than others, but it didn't stop me thinking to myself, 'Is somebody somewhere trying to tell me something?'

We had been in Churchdown only a matter of days when our first patient arrived. The news that a vet was in the village had spread quickly. This particular morning Angela answered the doorbell and was more than a little surprised to be confronted by a distraught lady with her injured spaniel. Despite the owner's attempts to stem the flow of blood from a leg wound, it continued to drip profusely through a combination of dressings, bandages and an old sock. We were unable to offer the benefits of a first-class operating theatre, which had yet to be set up, but with the benefit of Crudwell-style veterinary ingenuity we could sort the problem out. What we needed was an operating table, clean surgical drapes, a nurse and a surgeon. Angela was thrown in at the deep end as usual and her vet nursing duties commenced in the lounge. She suggested an old family wooden chest would make a temporary operating table, which she covered in a clean white sheet.

I wish I could remember the name of that dog, but Spaniel patient number 1 was soon heavily sedated with an injection of acetyl promazine, the area surrounding his deep lacerated wound was anaesthetised with local anaesthetic, and the traumatised area washed and cleansed with saline and the iodine-based pevidene. The surgery was straightforward; tie off the exuding blood vessels, remove tissues that were no longer viable and close the wound using only healthy tissues. Not bad for front-room surgery. The sutures were removed ten days later and all was well once more.

We hoped the successful treatment of our first patient, albeit in unconventional surroundings, would provide a little of the word-of-mouth advertising that was acceptable to our governing body. It later became permissible to have an illuminated sign fixed to the surgery wall displaying the words 'veterinary surgeon'. The purpose of the sign was, of course, to assist people who had been there before in identifying the practice on a dark winter evening, and not to advertise it to anyone that had not. The size of the letters could be no larger than one inch tall and lit by a background bulb no more than 25 Watts.

It was a mixed blessing. The relaxation of the rules was a start and most practices took advantage of it, although it was soon considered a waste of time. In reality anyone with good eyesight would still require a telescope to find it. One practitioner wrote to the *Veterinary Record* pointing out that in his area the small sign was causing confusion to the general public and after a few weeks they had taken it down. The staff of his practice had become fed up with explaining to people with bursting bladders that their waiting room was not a public convenience.

For us nothing could have been worse than the 'Churchdown Widow' saga. Elderly Mrs Gough and her family of cats had become a regular client of the practice in a very short space of time. She did not live far from the surgery and often called in for a chat about her cats. This informality was welcomed and never considered a waste of anyone's professional time. However, with the worst of bad luck Mrs Gough did not really have to struggle for reasons to visit the surgery. In one short spell she had lost two of her cats due to serious terminal illnesses. Sadly I had put to sleep one suffering from chronic renal failure and another with incurable feline leukaemia. To add to her woes, Mrs Gough was met one morning by a third cat dragging himself up her garden path. One of his front legs was so severely traumatised that surgical treatment and amputation of the leg was necessary. Mrs Gough feared the worst and believed she was about to lose another member of her family. The seriousness of the situation was explained to her. 'If you can save him, Mr Smith, please do whatever you have to.'

At that time I felt one of those 'special occasion' operations was required, not one that required exceptional surgical skills, but where success and a full recovery was essential. I operated that day. The surgery went well and I believed he would make a good recovery. Cats are remarkable animals at adapting quickly to life on three legs. Shortly after we received a telephone call from a reporter at a local newspaper who had heard of the unfortunate fate of Mrs Gough's three cats. He telephoned during a busy Saturday morning surgery and apologised for bothering me. We chatted for a couple of minutes and as usual from the outset I stressed to him that if I was to be quoted at all then there must be no possibility that I could be personally identified from my comments. He of course gave me that assurance, before asking me,

'Can you confirm that Mrs Gough has lost two of her cats in as many weeks and a third one has received grotesque injuries?'

'Yes, very sadly she has', I replied sympathetically. 'She has had a dreadful run of unbelievable misfortune.'

'A bit of a coincidence, isn't it?' Our reporter asked. 'Do you think someone could have a vendetta against Mrs Gough?' He was so eager for a story his imagination was running riot. 'Thank you so much for your time, Mr Smith.' The line went dead.

I carried on with morning surgery and thought no more of the telephone conversation until Monday evening. I went home at the end of surgery. It wasn't far to go as I lived next door of course, but usually by the time I got in at 7.30, and often much later, the children were in bed and it had been left to Angela to read their bedtime stories. On this particular evening I was greeted by a worried-looking wife and, 'Ive, I think you may have a big problem.'

She was still reading the headlines of the local newspapers. The most dramatic referred to the butchering of a local widow's cat. A touching picture of Mrs Gough and one of her cats had made front-page news. The first short paragraph related to her distress and the tragedies of the three cats, which the story suggested must be connected. The following paragraphs and almost the rest of the front page appeared to relate to my 'belief' that the three cases were related to the reporter's vendetta theory. It was of course 'just too much to be coincidence, wasn't it?' No it blooming well wasn't. But the seeds of doubt had been sown.

The reporter didn't go quite so far as to suggest that there was a maniac on the loose with a hatchet, but he had gone too far for the likes of the Royal College. Suddenly we were involved with solicitors to get our version of events in quickly before I was hauled up before the disciplinarians. Letters of explanation and apology were sent to the various divisions of the British Veterinary Society, and, more importantly, to local practitioners. Explanations to the latter were probably unnecessary. My relationship with the neighbouring practices was always sound. We were a small profession who enjoyed the occasional dig at each other, but faced with a serious problem we were united.

'There but for the grace of God go I.' We were all too familiar with this philosophical quip for a multitude of reasons. One cheeky prominent local veterinary practitioner did ring up to remind me that I had forgotten to give the reporter my telephone number. We are still very good friends. It sounds ridiculous now that something so frivolous should have caused so much worry and stress at the time.

It was a wonderful feeling having your own practice and knowing that you were running your own business, whichever way round you put it, even if you were not earning enough to make a living, but it was also a very stressful time. There were occasions when the enormity of what I had set out to do struck home. Among the considerations there was a huge mortgage, a wife, a child and another on the way to support. I tried not to think about it too often.

In order to succeed I needed patients, the trust of my clients and clinical results. In other words the people who brought their animals to me wanted to see them get better quickly. Putting up one's plate can be a lonely world without other colleagues in the practice to discuss your cases with. Even now I reflect on some early cases that perhaps did not go terribly wrong, but which did not go terribly well either. I am probably being a little paranoid but I still remember a couple of cases I wish had turned out differently.

To have got our diagnosis right most of the time without modern aids required considerable skill and experience, and it was quite an achievement, even if we say it ourselves. Many vet practices at that time did not even have basic X-ray facilities, or if they had, the poor quality radiographs they produced were often of no diagnostic value. The thorough basic clinical examination of the pet was essential. More often than not the thermometer, stethoscope and your own senses were the only available diagnostic tools.

I do not think this would have influenced the outcome of the young Labrador that was presented in surgery one morning. His vomiting had worsened over several days and after I had examined him one thing was certain: a rapid exploratory laparotomy of his abdomen was a priority. Everywhere the abdomen was palpated the digestive tract felt abnormal. Every inch of gut seemed to be in a contracted spasm. An X-ray would not have influenced the treatment, but it would have been a great help in convincing the owners from the start of the seriousness of the situation. The puppy did not survive the operation.

In different circumstances and with a successful outcome this particular case would still be talked about today, probably with some hilarity. On this occasion I did not want to talk about it. Several days earlier the pup had obviously rummaged through one of his owner's bedrooms and, of all the things he had found to eat, he had chosen a pair of ladies' elastic tights. The result was a surgical nightmare. The main body of the tights had remained in the stomach while, over the next few days, the leg parts gradually extended through the intestinal tract beyond. The vomiting, dehydration, pain and shock caused by the garment were overwhelming.

I had not really recovered from the disappointment of this case and could not believe things could get worse for a young vet trying to impress. But, good or bad, things do seem to run in twos and threes, and it was not long before Jasper became ill. This Jack Russell terrier also had an obsession for eating anything he could get his mouth around and there seemed to be no limit to his voracious appetite. It was simply a matter of time before he met with serious trouble, probably surgical. One day he was brought to morning surgery vomiting and bloated from a mainly bone-impacted bowel and showing the usual signs of dehydration and weakness that so frequently complicate these situations. Enemas had little effect on his impaction and clearly, if he was to be relieved of this very serious condition, surgery was required. I carried out the preliminary laparotomy but, to my horror and dismay, within a short time Jasper gave up the fight and died on the operating table.

When operating on an animal today – be it Joe Bloggs' old cat or the Queen's corgies – the owner would make no difference to me at all in the way that I made my clinical decisions. But at that time how I wished that Jasper had not been owned by Fred Stevens. In the short time we had been in Churchdown I was familiar with few names, but Mr Stevens was one of them. He seemed to be involved in everything in the Churchdown community, knew everyone, owned an awful lot of property, and was clearly a very able businessman. I rang Mr Stevens and said I would like to come round and speak with him. There has never been any doubt in my mind that he knew exactly the reason for my call.

I rang the door bell and immediately the front door opened. We sat facing each other in the lounge. I did not really know what to expect. Naturally I feared the worst – that he would suggest I leave Churchdown as soon as possible. I shall remember the next few minutes of conversation all my life. It was unexpected. Of course he was saddened that I had not been able to save his beloved dog, but he did not blame me in any way for that and accepted without hesitation that I had done my best for Jasper. Among other complimentary comments, he was impressed that, despite the lack of expectation, I had made an effort to meet and talk to him, knowing full well that it would have been easier to have quickly explained away the sad events in a telephone call. Some good things do arise from adversity and I left his house with a feeling of renewed confidence.

Today we, or at least the Health and Safety Executive, would no doubt be more concerned with the way we were running our veterinary practice than the routines of those early days. They would probably be having convulsions now, but despite our shortcomings we survived.

On a very limited budget there was no opportunity for the installation of expensive safeguards, even if they had been available. Initially, Mrs Farlow's kitchen was ideally placed to become the maid of all work, perhaps described today as a multi-functional room. It was equipped with a sturdy examination table complete with a heavy lead-surface mat just in case you ever wanted to use it for an X-ray of a patient – which we soon would – as well as the essential anaesthetic machine. It was amazing what could be fitted into such a small space. After morning surgery the consulting room rapidly transormed into the operating theatre.

For most of that first year a typical morning would find me standing by the operating table dressed in the traditional green surgeon's robes. My wife raised the sedated cat or dog's prominent cephalic leg vein, I steadily injected the induction dose of thiopentone and the animal relaxed and obligingly went to sleep. The mouth was opened wide. In went the endotracheal tube and the patient was connected to the gaseous halothane anaesthetic machine.

Angela had already sterilised the surgical instruments in the reliable 'fish kettle' for twenty minutes. This was an elongated stainless steel receptacle with a lid and a removable perforated tray. It was suitable and efficient for sterilising most of the instruments and soft materials such as swabs but it had one big disadvantage: for an infuriating length of time the instruments were too hot to handle! The pet had been clipped, the operation site cleaned, sterilised and draped. The operation could began.

Operations during those early years of the practice were certainly family affairs. Somehow we managed to fit in the requirements of a one-year-old son who had a ringside seat to observe veterinary surgery from his highchair. We developed a satisfactory routine and as usual when you are enjoying yourself time seems to go much more quickly. The months passed by too fast and my pregnant wife/nurse was standing increasingly further away from the operating table. When it became clear that Angela's arms were no longer able to reach the patient comfortably we placed an advertisement in the local press for our first nurse/receptionist employee.

We were overwhelmed with replies, but I knew that with just one vacancy, many local applicants would be disappointed, and some would be really disgruntled. It was the sort of feeling that I had when asked to judge a dog show or an exhibit at a WI meeting. I felt that when the winner was announced I was about to meet one person who appreciated my brilliance in these matters and fifty more who believed I was stupid anyway. I am sure I was just being unnecessarily paranoid.

The job was offered to Pat, a bright and vivacious young lady who was leaving Chosen Hill School with a large handful of very good O-level results. She was certainly well qualified to be our nurse/receptionist. The practice grew rapidly and it was satisfying to be able to offer jobs to others. Pat remained with the practice for many years before she married and moved to Cornwall. By then, as she frequently reminded me, her job description should really have been head nurse/receptionist/cleaner/secretary/practice manager/radiographer.

Actually, when Pat first started, we didn't do any radiography; we could not afford the expensive X-ray machine. Buying the machine was a huge financial investment for a small business still trying to get off the ground. It is unimaginable now to think that it cost just a little short of half of what we paid for the whole premises. It was financed via the manager of Cheltenham's Montpellier branch of the Midland Bank, Mr White. He did not look like Captain Mainwaring, but our business relationship I suspect was similar to that of our *Dad's Army* hero.

'Ivor, you can borrow as much as you like', he said, with our house deeds safely tucked away in his strongroom, 'but don't find yourself in a position where you end up working every day for the Midland Bank.' I had tremendous respect for this man. It was a bit like talking to a favourite uncle whom I think had a genuine interest and regard for my practice, and right from the start his advice was sound. How that traditional customer/manager relationship would change in such a short time. Two decades later our bank manager was a spotty youth and we questionned whose side he was even on.

I ordered a state-of-the-art X-ray machine, the GEC MX-2. The descriptive brochures claimed that it was a portable unit that could be dismantled quickly and transported in your car for use on the farm or in a stable. In reality the farthest our machine ever travelled was the surgery drive to X-ray the legs of lame horses. By the time the machine had been disassembled in the surgery, reassembled on the surgery drive, used for ten minutes then disassembled, moved back into the surgery and then reassembled in time to take a quick radiograph of the most recently injured cat, you certainly did not need to visit the gym that day. It is a superb piece of medical equipment, but I still question its portability. It was distributed by an entrepreneurial gentleman named Edward Elston, whom I believe was based in Sussex and was the UK's sole distributor. Business was booming for him at the time and he travelled around the country delivering and setting up these machines from John O'Groats to Lands End. If the installation and staff instruction ran into a second day, Mr Elston overcame the issue of overnight accommodation by delivering the equipment in his large powerful car and towing a caravan, which on this occasion was easily accommodated on our practice drive. At the end of surgery that day, and following the initial staff tuition in radiography, we naturally invited him to join us for supper.

It was a jovial evening and the three-course *cordon bleu* supper Angela had prepared was accompanied by bottles of Chablis and Châteauneuf du Pape. While Angela served coffee and I poured the brandies, I happened to mention that it was unfortunate that Mr Elston's wife, at home in Sussex, was unable to be with us tonight.

'Oh, she's all right out there.'

'Out where?'

'Out in our caravan.'

'Which caravan?'

'The one on your drive', he replied quite casually. 'She enjoys a bit of knitting and likes reading her magazines.'

'Well, let's take her a cup of coffee', I offered, in utter disbelief.

'Oh no, no need to bother with that, she'll have her head down by now.'

An hour later her merry husband wobbled down the drive to rejoin her.

By the end of surgery the next morning the Elstons were back on the road and travelling on to the next practice, the next sale and, presumably, another sole supper. I never did have the opportunity to meet Mrs Elston. Her husband clearly ran a very successful business machine, and the machine he sold was even more successful. They were installed from one end of the country to the other. Thirty-five years later our original MX-2 was still in regular use, and still producing superb radiographs.

Who would have thought that so many intelligent pets could possibly eat those pins, needles, golf balls, undigested chop bones and all manner of unmentionable objects that we described to incredulous owners? Their X-rays were often spectacular and thanks are overdue to Mrs Elston for her part in delivering that machine. Her knitting, patience and tolerance have undoubtedly saved the lives of hundreds of animals.

I had never had any formal training on how to run a business and the technique I mainly used was to make it up as I went along. It was a fast learning curve but there were some early signs that I could indeed make a living running my own practice. I knew nothing at all about book-keeping but it wasn't long before I realised that this was an essential aspect of keeping things on an even keel. How fortunate I was to be able to call upon one of my old Crypt classmates, John Eggleton.

At the time I put up the plate John was employed by the accountants Deloittes from their Spa Road offices in Gloucester. We had lost track of each other since we had left school. John had left a couple of years before me to join his well-known family firm of accountants, and then I had left Gloucester to go to Liverpool. It was great to get back together and there was much to talk about. He came for an early supper one evening each week, and eventually we left Angela to look after the dishes while we moved to the surgery and the books. On most of those occasions we were still discussing bank statements, sales ledgers and all the paraphernalia of the records you were expected to keep for the benefit of the Inland Revenue, at midnight. It was still a few years before the VAT man arrived on the scene and thereafter the record keeping seemed to treble.

With a little help from my friends I must have been doing the right thing most of the time. The practice was growing quickly and within two to three years we needed a vet assistant. This made an unbelievably pleasant difference to our lives. Not working all the hours of the day, we were soon on the riverbanks fishing once again and enjoying times we had not experienced since we were teenagers.

John had become engaged to Jacqui and over the years we enjoyed many pleasant meals together in restaurants in Cheltenham and Gloucester. The Bistro Bacchus in Spa Road was one of our favourites at that time. In some ways it was ahead of its time and its popularity meant that we invariably bumped into other long-lost friends there. John had enjoyed a successful rugby career playing scrum-half for Longlevens, but he was also an excellent cricketer.

On one occasion we arranged to spend a Saturday evening at a dinner/dance at the Carlton Hotel in Cheltenham. These live band dances were very popular at that time and the disco had not yet arrived. You would not be allowed in without a jacket and tie but nevertheless we quite enjoyed wearing our dark suits. For me it made a pleasant change from my shirt and working jeans. We relaxed at the end of the meal and before the band struck up we lit our cigarettes. I find it difficult to believe now that we enjoyed a smoke, but at the time it was harder to find someone who did not. In sophisticated fashion I lifted the flickering candlestick and held it inches from John's face – he inhaled and the cigarette glowed. Then I tilted the candle towards me and in true James Bond fashion lit up. I have never seen melted candle wax drip on to the lap of 007. As it cooled on my smart trousers it turned white, and when I stood up Angela grimaced and as quietly as possible ordered me to 'Sit down!' If I had ventured on to the dance floor I would surely have been asked by the management staff to leave the premises immediately. Somehow I had to remove the adhering hard layer of glistening white wax. We came up with a cunning plan. I moved inconspicuously to the Gent's with my hands cupped in front of me, masking the affected area. John followed closely behind with a table knife. In the privacy of the toilet we got down to business. John volunteered to do the scraping so I sat on a chair and he took up a kneeling position with his back to the door and began scraping. Within minutes he was making good progress and I was beginning to feel more respectable and less fearful of someone misinterpreting the situation. But things were about to get a lot worse. The main door of the toilets flew open and none other than the manager entered. 'This is where we get ejected', I thought, with John's head closer to my lap than the damned candlestick ever was. His words were more than a little surprising.

'Oh, I am terribly sorry to have interrupted you gentlemen', he almost whispered and promptly disappeared back out the door. In disbelief, I looked down at John and John looked up at me. He took seconds to complete the job and we shot back out to the restaurant. We rejoined the ladies and were relieved to find security was not waiting for us.

There were some wonderful summers through the 1970s and some freaky weather as well. We were really too tied to the practice to go away on holiday, but it was not a terrible hardship to spend time in our huge garden. The pleasure came as much from designing, planting and generally working in the garden as sitting in it, and it was always a labour of love.

I recall watching the television news in May 1975; with dramatic warnings of hazardous driving conditions on some of the motorways due to heavy snowfall at the beginning of the week. By the end of that week, with the temperature in the high 70s, that year's heatwave had begun in most parts of the country.

The following year, 1976, was the year of the drought. The heat was astonishing that summer and it led to unexpected practical problems in the practice. The anaesthetic machine we used was very basic and, looking back, unbelievably primitive, even though when I had bought it a few years earlier it was considered to be state-of-the-art. The serious problem we faced was that the amount of vaporised halothane gas delivered to the patient increased rapidly with a rise in temperature, and none of us had experienced heat like this before. We now risked inadvertently administering an overdose of anaesthetic to our patients.

Fortunately, there was an easy solution. Well, easy I should say for the natural early risers, but a bit more difficult for the last-minute souls. We started operating before the sun rose, and for several weeks our operating sessions began before 6 o'clock, when the outside temperature was still around 80°F. It was too hot to sleep anyway. There were mornings when I was out and about on an urgent call at around 4 o'clock and many owners were already out walking their dog. Not surprisingly there weren't many joggers around.

For Angela and me the '70s had begun perilously, but had ended with us content and successful. From practically nothing the primitive practice had become a thriving veterinary centre in the rural area we loved, and we were providing veterinary care for a rapidly growing population. Our daughter, Sally, was one of them. She arrived in 1972 during the practice's first year and it was our privilege to ask John Eggleton to be her godfather. There could not have been a better choice.

The most memorable social occasion of the decade had to be the Royal celebrations of 1977. Despite a grave economic crisis at the time, in keeping with the rest of the country our village was determined to celebrate the Silver Jubilee of the Queen's accession in 1952 in style. Every British village would hold their own celebration and every inhabitant was involved.

Naturally there would be an old-fashioned farm tractor and trailer procession around the village of Churchdown with local costumed residents attempting to keep their balance on the back of the trailers. The decorative floats represented many different but related themes. Our float was 'Humpty Dumpty and all the King's Men'; it was great fun and all the participants were quite well behaved, compared to the last occasion I had ventured aboard.

That particular occasion had been about fifteen years ago and was part of Liverpool University's rag week panto procession. The first year students of each faculty were expected to produce the winning item. Twenty-eight of my red-blooded veterinary mates and six Boudiccas had then defended our mobile 'Lady Chatterley's Gamekeeper's Hut' from hundreds of marauding Scousers. On our trek around the streets of Liverpool there had been several unfortunate events. We sent flowers and apologies to make amends for one of them. At the time we passed a ladies' hairdressing salon, an attractive young Liverpudlian hairdresser ventured on to the pavement to watch the procession go by. We whisked her up on to our float and it was much later that we heard of the complaints of her customer, who had been left unattended under a hairdryer for a couple of hours.

There was no pillaging of our float in Churchdown, only the odd cheeky remark from bystanders to put up with. It turned out to be an overcast English summer's day, but a happy one, cheered by the numerous Union Jack flags flying everywhere.

I am sure many will have no difficulty remembering their ride on the 'elephant' in the company of 'zoo keeper' Uncle Adam Pullen. Adam and his brother Ben were accustomed to caring for hundreds of cattle at nearby Home Farm, however looking after one mechanical elephant for a few hours was quite a challenge. Angela had already met this wonderful beast, who was the star of the show at a children's party, just a couple of weeks before. When she asked if he was free on this special day the generous owners were more than delighted to deliver him to us from Cheltenham – not in a horse-box, but on a Bullinghams the Builders truck. With just a drop of oil and a couple of pints of petrol, his lawn mower power house worked well all day. Adam tired long before the elephant or the children did, having walked up and down a field a few hundred times. I was so pleased this animal required no medical attention. I might have ended up kicking a mower that wouldn't work.

Evening celebrations took place in a myriad of venues. We gathered post-procession in the grounds of Teviotdale, at that time the home of David and Jane Foyle. An outbuilding had been transformed into a traditional village alehouse. They had made such an impressive success of this that for many years afterwards the village children could not understand where that other pub in the village was.

The 1970s had been an immensely challenging but enjoyable decade for us. But the river of life does not always run smoothly; now and again in the next decade the river would become quite turbulent.

CHAPTER SIX

LIFE BEGINS AT FORTY

Ido not know for sure who conjured up the cliché 'life begins at forty', but I recall thinking a great deal about it each time my birthday came round while in my thirties. I remember the tune being whistled or hummed by my parents whilst as a youngster, and I know that it was a well-known song recorded in 1937 by Sophie Tucker. I have no idea why I should remember this amazingly insignificant fact as I am hopeless at Trivial Pursuit. One fact I do remember well is my date of birth, and my staff rarely forgot it either. They were so keen to celebrate in fact, that they even jumped the gun and celebrated my fortieth a year early.

It was a little embarrassing at the time, but their generosity and wit was appreciated. The appropriately rude birthday card, the candles, cake and bottle of Phyllosan tablets (the essential pills to fortify the over forties), appeared, and even a small bottle of champagne. There was an awkward moment's silence when I tactfully suggested they check my year of birth. On doing so, they apologised for their error, sang 'Happy Birthday', and drank the champers anyway.

Three hundred and sixty-five days later they did it all again, this time presenting me with a bigger bottle of Phyllosan. Then they drank a bigger bottle of champers.

The 1970s passed quickly. Veterinary assistants came and went, gained experience with us and then moved on. The day-to-day running of veterinary practice life revolved around Anne, Rosemary and Debbie. Individually it would have been hard to select three more different people but we bonded well and formed the nucleus of a happy and successful team. In a small business and in the pre-specific job description days, there was frequently overlap, but no one complained.

Anne was the practice secretary. She and her husband hailed from the Forest of Dean, although they had been part of the vibrant Churchdown community for many years. They had both been educated at Lydney Grammar School, the scene of many rugby battles in which I had taken part. That was at a time when their school seemed capable of producing far more than its fair share of schoolboy international players. Trevor Wintle, Cledwyn and John Davies, and Bev Dovey are names that come quickly to mind. I was fortunate enough to have had the opportunity to play against them, when we usually lost, and with them, as Gloucestershire schoolboys, when we usually won.

Where Anne was chatty and pleasantly flamboyant, Rosemary was particularly quiet and a little reserved, but a confident and professional nurse. Her slim stature was deceptive and she was a tough nut who never seemed to tire. She went home when the day's work had been completed to her satisfaction and everything had been prepared for an early start the next morning. Rosemary had joined the practice in response to our advertisement in the *Veterinary Record* for a qualified RANA, one of our 'girls in green' whom we trusted and respected. She moved from London to take up the position.

Interviews often seem to be predictable, but on this occasion I was taken a little by surprise. Those were the days when the practice was expected to provide accommodation for both veterinary and nursing staff, and at the time it was unusual to be asked if there were any objections to the nurse's partner sharing the accommodation. This now sounds naïvely prudish, but attitudes and expectations have changed significantly in thirty years. I could see no reason why I should object. Actually there was a very good reason: can you believe this – her boyfriend played in the front row for Wasps! It might have been worse of course, he could have been a Bath player. Now if ever there was chalk and cheese. He was a lovely guy off the field, and no doubt the diminutive Rosemary felt secure when she disappeared into the arms of her London prop forward.

Debbie was an enigma. She represents a type of staff member present in probably most of the veterinary practices throughout the country. For various reasons she hadn't obtained the formal qualifications to study to become a qualified veterinary nurse, but as a result of her association with vets and nurses within the practice over the years, she had become an extremely knowledgeable and invaluable asset, familiar with anaesthetic procedures and someone we could trust. After many years she eventually left The Brambles practice to take up a career in the clinical environment of an NHS hospital laboratory, a post to which she was more than suitably qualified. The clients missed her caring attention and I missed her dry sense of humour.

Debbie had been part of the practice for just a few weeks and was on duty over the Christmas period. There had been a dreadful accident on Boxing Day. Early in the afternoon a speeding car had mounted the pavement and struck a group of people on Innsworth Lane. There had been several fatalities, including a patient of ours, a large German Shepherd dog.

At the time of the tragedy, we had been enjoying the seasonal company of Old Cryptians and Old Richians at their Longlevens rugby club. Traditionally for many, this was the festive day of Christmas when the teams of grammar school old boys fought it out for the Horns Trophy. The post-match celebrations were the best local rugby had to offer, and continued late into the afternoon. For some they continued late into the evening, but at about 4 o'clock, most of the wives and girlfriends drove their happy warriors home.

Within minutes of arriving home Angela and I were aware that this was not how our Boxing Day was normally concluded. Immediately I was in sobering discussions with emergency service officers. They quickly explained all that had happened and I arranged for our duty vet and a nurse to attend the scene of the carnage. It was a dreadful way to end such an enjoyable day, and difficult to remove the pictures of what had happened from my mind. We sat zombie-like in front of the television while Morecambe and Wise did their best to cheer us up.

The following day it was back to business. At 8.30 a.m. I wandered round the surgery trying rapidly to catch up with all the important events that had happened in my absence. It was customary for any unfortunate creature that we had put to sleep to be placed in a thick black plastic bag before being transferred to the confines of a chest freezer. Lifting the body of a large dog – literally a dead weight – into the freezer was often physically impossible for a nurse to undertake on her own. I assumed that one of the black bags contained the Boxing Day tragedy, so I casually asked, 'What's in the other bag, Debbie?'

'Oh, that's the other half of the dog, Mr Smith' she replied innocently. I gulped.

For most people buying a freezer should be nothing more strenuous than a trip to a nearby high-street chain. Normally you would just hope that there would be sufficient funds on the credit card to cover the cost of the purchase. That is unless you are a vet.

Needing a new appliance for the surgery, our visit to the local branch of electrical goods started well and we were pleased to be greeted by the shop assistant who just happened to be a Brockworth lady we knew well; she was the devoted owner of miniature Poodles and a frequent visitor to our surgery. Half an hour later things were not going so well. She was determined not to sell me a chest freezer and continued to try and convince me that we needed the more economical modern one with five sliding drawers. At the peak of my frustration I resisted the temptation to ask her, 'How the hell do I get a Rottweiler into one of those?' At the end of an awkward and protracted debate I bought a big chest freezer anyway and no doubt left my client hoping I would fall into it! Thankfully, she remained a loyal client whom I saw frequently. We talked about ear infections, itchy skin and the weather, but never about fridges.

Farm practice at this time was immensely enjoyable, and at that time I could not get enough of it. I was young and fit enough still to relish the challenge of the cold wet weather, the mud, the kicks and the physical effort needed to calve cows. There was still opportunity too to practise farm animal medicine the way we had been taught at Liverpool.

A short distance out of Churchdown, travelling towards Brockworth, was Woodhouse Farm. At the time, the Davies, a lovely elderly Welsh couple lived and in a small way farmed there. Early one afternoon the practice received a call from a very worried Mr Davies asking if I would be kind enough to visit him as soon as possible to see a calf that was fitting.

None of the calves in the group looked particularly well and the one that had prompted the visit was indeed showing neurological signs, frothing at the mouth and staggering around the small concrete yard. The poor beast was grinding his teeth and within minutes of my arrival collapsed and died.

The list of possible different causes flashed through my mind. Was this a case of a bacterial infection, listeriosis or tetanus? A nutritional disorder was possible, so was cerebrocortical necrosis of the brain, magnesium deficiency, or even poisoning. I found myself rattling off the list of possibilities that not so long ago I was repeating like poetry to my Liverpool Vet School lecturers.

I hung my hat on this being a case of lead poisoning. I was alarmed when Mr Davies told me that a calf in the group had died a couple of days earlier. On closer examination, all the calves were showing the early signs of the illness – the teeth grinding and the abdominal pain. I took a couple of blood samples to check for the presence of lead, but if these animals were to be saved then I had to act immediately. I slipped back to the surgery and collected bottles of calcium versonate and, returning to the farm, injected each of the calves intravenously. They had more the next day and they recovered. I arranged for a post-mortem examination to be carried out at the ever-helpful Veterinary Investigation Centre at Elmbridge Court, and there my diagnosis was confirmed from the flakes of blue paint found in the calve's rumen, and later from the high levels of lead in the blood samples.

The diagnosis was not rocket science. It had not taken long to find where the calves had obtained the lead. An old door, among other items, had been used as a wall to confine the cattle, and calves do have an obsession with licking things; in this instance that included the peeling door paint. Today of course paint does not normally contain lead and this once common problem is thankfully now a rarity. Farmers are traditionally versatile in transforming old doors into new objects and there were many of them in use at another neighbouring farm, a little closer to Churchdown.

Harry and Barbara Hopton farmed at Woodfield Farm. The farm buildings are situated on one side of the old narrow Brockworth road and the farmhouse, which has a distinctive pattern of chequered red brick, is on the opposite side. The couple were a brother and sister team and despite their constant arguing ran the farm well. It is difficult to describe Harry. He looked an old chap when I first met him in the 1960s, and looked no different thirty years later. Wearing his distinctive NHS wire spectacles he could well have been Albert Steptoe's twin brother. Barbara was a lovely country lady who for many years rode her bike around the village.

Harry walked everywhere. I do not know whether this was because he believed it more economical or because he could not ride a bike. He did not have a telephone and getting in touch with him meant visiting him at home; this could be tricky. Having knocked on the front door, which was at the side of the building, reaching the hub of the house – the farm kitchen – entailed running the gauntlet past the most vicious little Jack Russell, which was usually tied to a table leg in the scullery. He would dive at your leg as you tried to get past while Barbara prodded him with a walking stick and told him to behave himself.

Like Harry, some farmers at that time were notoriously cheeky when it came to paying their bills. The usual routine was to pull out the vet's bill that was tucked under the wireless set, squint at the bottom line and wince. The bill and cheque-book were then handed over with the request, 'I expect you'd like to fill this in yourself, Mr Smith, and don't forget some good luck money.' The idea of course was that the bill would be rounded down plus a bit more, and after I had checked that it was the last bill he had been sent, that is of course what I did. Today we call it discount if it is paid on time!

Driving to Brockworth Court Farm one morning, I was surprised to see an agitated Harry on the road attempting to run towards Churchdown. He was waving his hands in the air and shouting something. I had to stop to avoid hitting him.

'Quick, Vet', he yelled, 'I need 'elp to get a bullock out of a trough that's stuck upside down with his arse in the air.' I returned to the farm gates with him. The reason for his panic was easy enough to spot – with four long bovine legs pointing up and not down. We began to walk calmly through the other twenty-odd cattle that were part of the group when suddenly, in the midst of the milling cattle, I spotted Barbara, sitting battered and bruised among them on the ground, covered in everything the farmyard had to offer.

'Hang on a minute, Harry', I said. 'What's going on here?'

'Ne'r moind 'bout 'er, we gotta get this bugger outa 'ere.'

'We're going to get Barb out first', I stated.

Attracted by the amount of unusual activity as he passed by, John Halford could not have arrived at a more opportune time. We carried a distressed Barbara to safety and left Harry swearing at his upside-down steer. We left Barbara in her favourite kitchen chair, nipped back to the farmyard, turned the water trough and its contents over and freed the beast. He was suffering from loss of dignity and a bit of bruising but it was clear that Barbara's injuries were more serious. We ignored her 'Oh, I'll be all right' pleas and called for an ambulance. The trampling cattle had fractured her pelvis and a femur. She was a tough nut and, happily, a few months and a couple of major operations later, she was back on the farm and back on her bike.

As the years went by she and Harry did make some efforts to move into the twentieth century and a new indoor toilet was installed. It was not one that was joined up to a sewage system, but a cesspit was a vast improvement and it was no longer necessary to take a trip to the little building at the end of the garden. I have no recollection of them ever having a telephone put into the house, but eventually they did invest in a television set and at last they were able to see a world that existed beyond Churchdown.

Geoff Saxon lived on a small farm named Windermere at Bamfurlong, a hamlet between Churchdown and Cheltenham. I cannot remember the first time I met this workaholic but I should. He was from the north-east and fortunately had an accent that we could understand and a wonderful sense of humour. I never asked him how he got into farming or how he came to be in our neck of the woods, but perhaps it was better that I hadn't. He was mainly interested in cattle and pigs and they were well cared for, though sometimes not in a well-organised way. As well as farming with his son, Paul, they owned and drove very large transport wagons. Geoff really needed a twenty-five-hour day to fit in all that he did, and he often looked in want of it.

I usually met Mrs Saxon when I visited the farm and it was to Sue that I could most relate. There were frequent differences of opinion between them when I was on the farm but happily they were usually resolved while I was still there. Geoff's northern humour shone through in adversity, and on those occasions when it was necessary to break a silence, usually after I had pinched my fingers for the third time in the rusting latches of his cattle crush, tuberculin testing his wild Charollais cows, he was still able to remark, 'Bet it isn't like this at Pullens.' It wasn't, but I never laboured the point. He was referring to his big farming neighbour, where things were indeed organised a little differently – albeit with a lot more help. Nevertheless he provided the fun and the stories. One Sunday morning found him on the farm sawing logs with a circular saw. He must have been distracted at the time he ripped through the thumb on his right hand.

'Christ, I've sawn my bloody thumb off!' he yelled. Sue knew that Geoff was prone to exaggeration and shouted back, 'Don't you be so silly!' He held his hand aloft and on this occasion she believed him and put the box of plasters away.

Within the hour they had reached the Accident and Emergency Department at Gloucester's Hospital, accompanied by a couple of local farm-working pals. He was quickly referred to a specialist surgeon, who was no doubt looking forward to a couple of challenging hours of reconstructive surgery. Asked if they had brought the missing digit with them, the lads apologised and said they would go back and look for it. Half an hour later they were back with the main portion of the thumb. The surgeon cast his eye over the adhering sawdust, various samples of animal faeces and other unrecognisable things. He made his mind up instantly and decided it was in Geoff's best interest to go ahead and amputate the remnant of his thumb.

It was not the end of the world for Geoff, but losing the thumb of your best hand could lead to a lifetime of frustration for any farmer. Apart from anything else, farmers needed that thumb to 'nose' cattle. The largest of cattle could usually be controlled with a good armlock and a firm index finger and thumb pinching with the other strong arm. It drove Geoff mad when he could no longer do it. It drove me mad when he let go and I was thumped by the cow he was supposed to be restraining.

There was an occasion when another neighbour's saddleback gilts were running with a group of Geoff's large white gilts with reputedly the best large white boar in the county. We had some of the best pig farms in the country not so very far away. Time had gone by and if a gilt was pregnant she would be by now and for husbandry reasons the neighbouring farmer wanted his pigs back.

The problem was the weather. It would not stop raining, and this led to a further problem – mud, glorious mud. The irate neighbour demanded his pigs back. An equally irate and frustrated Geoff said he could not have them.

'Look, until it stops raining there's bugger all I can do. I can't sort 'em out. I don't know whether they are supposed to be my white pigs or your black and white pigs or someone else's black pigs. They are all black pigs and they all look the bloody same to me.' No doubt the only person not frustrated at the time was the large white boar, whatever colour he happened to be at that time.

A few miles away, as you approach Gloucester from the direction of Stroud, you descend the steep Birdlip Hill and to your left you see through the trees the beautiful views of Witcombe Lakes. They appear to be natural lakes but they are of course relatively modern reservoirs. Everything else, however, is the wonderful countryside that would have been enjoyed by our Roman ancestors. I really began to appreciate the true beauty of this area on my frequent visits to Mr Metson, who farmed at the picturesque Coopers Hill Farm. I am sure that there must be scores of local people who can still remember Mr Metson the milkman. He was a milk producer/retailer who delivered the early morning pints and quarts to homes in Brockworth and Hucclecote from churns in his pony and trap.

The telephone rang shortly after 5 o'clock one fine June morning. Most farmers start the telephone conversation with an honest apology. Then there are others who open the conversation with, 'I'm glad you are up already and I haven't disturbed you, Ivor.' There were occasions when I would have loved to say with some truth, 'Actually, I have only just got into bed.'

Mr Metson's description of his cow needing an early morning call was the last thing you wanted to hear before you had properly woken up, but it was an emergency. A prolapse of the uterus is not an uncommon complication in a cow suffering from milk fever shortly after calving. The calcium deficiency leads to a loss in muscle tone and the continued straining sometimes allows the uterus to invert and the vast organ simply turns inside out.

'I'll be with you shortly, but get as many towels under her womb as you can.' The last thing we needed was further damage to the uterus from Cotswold weeds and thistles. As so often happens, the cow had collapsed to the ground with her head uphill, allowing gravity to ensure the prolapse was complete. Even without the morning's first mug of tea, I found the energy to rope and swing her hind legs in the opposite direction, carefully manoeuvring the prolapsed organ with her.

Gravity is one of life's mysteries and there are times like this when it is a very welcome force working in your favour. Twenty minutes later, with my patient's head pointing downhill, the one hundredweight of inverted uterus was returned to its rightful place. This very important organ had naturally suffered an immense amount of superficial damage and in the short term she would need treatment for a transient uterine infection, but with the appropriate attention she would probably breed again. I cannot say for sure but I like to think that she did.

Within minutes of the routine intravenous calcium treatment, mum was back on her feet and her calf's head was pummeling at the udder and enjoying her morning milk. I declined Mr Metson's offer of early morning coffee and, stripped to the waist, scrubbed myself as clean as I could in the fresh morning air, enjoying the wondrous views of green fields and surrounding majestic hills that lay in all directions. Tucked away in this mysterious place are the remains of Witcombe's Roman villa. There isn't really a lot for the tourist to see but to the historian it's intriguing. Some experts suggest that at some time there was a much larger and more important Roman villa in the area, the ruins of which are still waiting to be unearthed.

Mr Metson eventually retired and in the 1970s Mark and Celia moved into Coopers Hill Farm. Mark Hicks-Beach was the owner of the Witcombe Park Estates, and lands as far as the Roman eye would have seen. In a short period of time he became one of my practice's largest farm clients and, in an equally short time, a close friend. Naturally there were a number of farming families with whom Angela and I developed close friendly relationships, and visiting their farms was a pleasurable bonus. Mark and his family were one of them. To me he had all those special qualities that I admire in being British, and some, if I am honest, I envied.

Mark was Eton educated, outwardly inspiring and confident and a very good organiser. He blended well with his band of farm staff who I am certain had great respect for him. During the working day it was fascinating to listen to the usual farm banter but in the contrasting tones of a distinctive Oxford accent and that of broad Gloucestershire all in harmony. His commonsense and natural organising ability made him an excellent local politician, and for many years he served as a Tewkesbury borough councillor. Mark accepted his limitations and he knew how to delegate. But here's a secret. He had a phobia of flying. He hated it so much that on some family holidays he would meet up with Celia and the children by sea a few days later.

Back down to earth were the farmers and the folks who spent their whole life working on the farm. Many of my ancestors were simply described as agricultural labourers but I hope that they were as invaluable to the success of the running of their farms as so many of the loyal characters that I have had the pleasure to work with. Throughout my professional career there have been countless occasions when my job would have been very difficult, and at times impossible, without the company of the professional farmworker whose only qualifications were an abundance of common sense, a natural affinity with the animals and years of experience

Farm life at Witcombe would certainly have been less interesting without Arnold and Hubert. There is little that I need say about Arnold other than he was a very likeable, helpful and dependable member of staff. Hubert was a little different. Not so many years before, when we were at war with Nazi Germany, Hubert had been a member of Dad's Army and officially one of a group of part-time soldiers manning an anti-aircraft gun on the top of Birdlip Hill.

I find it difficult to describe Hubert. Such a likeable person could have been any one of television's *Dad's Army*, other than Captain Mainwaring, whom he definitely was not. He freely and bravely admitted that they would have defended to the last man the Cheeserollers, the Twelve Bells, the Royal George and the Royal William. There were probably other pubs a bit further a field where they played darts and there too they were prepared to make their last stand.

Not so very far away along the A46 towards Cheltenham was another farming client, John Ganley at Hunts Court Farm. The evidence of a German Messerschmitt fighter attack on the farm can still be seen today:

the imprints of the machine-gun fire pockmark the walls in abundance. I do not know why this German pilot swerved away from the aircraft factories at Brockworth to attack cattle and sheep at Shurdington. Perhaps he had got wind that our ace anti-aircraft gunner Hubert and his men were defending the local skies.

I remember Hubert's proclamation of intent to protect the pubs well (a big mature bullock was standing on my foot at the time), but I better remember the day we were tuberculin testing cattle at Coopers Hill Farm. For whatever reason, things were not going particularly well and our patience and vocabulary was being stretched. Perhaps the cattle had been through the cattle crush once too often recently for other farm husbandry procedures. It was certainly the wrong day to receive a visit from a disgruntled European tourist wanting to explore the remains of the Roman villa.

'Who the 'ell's this?' Hubert questioned, as a huge black saloon car approached menacingly up the farm drive. A large, smartly dressed balding man emerged from the shiny Mercedes.

'I am looking for a Roman villa and all we can find are some stones in a field', the guttural voice announced. 'Bloody 'ell, it's a German', Hubert remarked. Our visitor's next few words were highly critical of our useless tourist industry and advice on how we should avoid deceiving people. We thought his criticism was a little inappropriate.

'Shall I tell him to piss off?' Hubert asked Mark. Mark was far too diplomatic. After further aggravating comments I felt that one of us would have to challenge the man. Irritated, I put my tuberculin testing syringes to one side on a straw bale and turned to him.

'Look sir, there was a time when the Roman villa here was quite a big place, but one night on their way back home from Coventry the Luftwaffe flew over, chucked a few spares out, and flattened it.'

There was a brief moment of silence.

I got the impression he was not deeply impressed by my comments. He muttered something, probably not terribly flattering, to the other occupants of the Mercedes, climbed back in and quickly disappeared down the drive. One hopes they enjoyed their visit to our wonderfully still intact Gloucester Cathedral, and we continued tuberculin testing our fractious English beasts.

'I was just about to tell him to frig off', said Hubert.

Mark telephoned early one morning to ask if I would go along and assist a young beef cow that was having trouble calving. He sounded dreadful: he was obviously suffering from an infection of some description. He asked me to call at the farmhouse where Celia would take me to where the labouring cow had gone down a couple of fields away. On arrival, I could see that Mark was very much under the weather: he was standing in the kitchen in his pyjamas with a mug of tea in his hand, looking for all the world as though he were advertising Beecham's Powders. I collected my gear from the back of my car and off we marched.

It was another fantastic late spring morning. There was a nip in the air but you knew it would soon become a very warm day. Hubert was standing guard with the patient when we reached him.

'Don't worry, young lady', I reassured the cow, watching her strong abdominal muscles straining and achieving nothing. 'We'll soon sort your problems out.' I stripped to the waist, shivering as the freezing cold rubber of the protective calving gown came into contact with my skin. We had carried buckets of hot water with us from the farm and soon the area surrounding the occasional appearance of a calf's foot was as clean and aseptic as it could be in these circumstances. My hand and arm disappeared into the depths of the cow's uterus exploring the extent of her obstetrical problems. The calf was not in an ideal position for delivery, but the postural defect should not take long to correct. One of the calf's legs was pointing backwards instead of forwards and the head was looking at it. These are quite common bovine obstetrical problems and are usually quickly corrected, except in those cases where the calf is exceptionally large and there is little room to manoeuvre. This was one of them.

Introducing ever-increasing amounts of obstetrical lubricants around the calf Hubert suggested that the spare pint of Castrol XL that he had in his car might be of some use. On this occasion we ignored him. By now my operative left hand was numb from the enormous pressure inside the uterus and it was the wrong time for smart remarks. 'Another quip like that, Hubert, and you'll get some lubricant where it might surprise you', I thought to myself. I refrained, and asked him politely to pass me one of the clean obstetrical ropes. Celia passed me a rope, which I somehow secured to the absent foot with senseless fingers. I had already repositioned the head and instructed my assistants to haul on the rope to draw up the leg to its rightful place while I protected the uterus from the calf's sharp hoof with a cupped hand. We were making good progress until suddenly the traction stopped.

'What's up?' I enquired.

'I'm getting covered in filth, that's what', Celia complained. She had come to assist me calve a cow dressed in a white designer blouse and a floral skirt. 'Just give me a half a minute.' I did, and she unbuttoned her blouse and handed it to Hubert for safekeeping.

With the calf in the correct position and the ropes attached to both forelimbs, I was able to guide the head through that important canal. More spirited traction and the calf would emerge safely. At a critical moment there was another adjournment and everything stopped. The floral skirt was now getting covered in a mixture of foetal fluids and lubricants. Celia was not happy.

'I don't believe this', I thought to myself, as her skirt disappeared in the same direction as her blouse. With me hauling on one rope and Celia on the other, now looking like a model for Gossard lingerie, the calf at last lunged forward, safe and well. With our bovine patient and her new calf secure in Hubert's safe hands, we returned to the farmhouse.

I had removed my calving gown – now plastered in every conceivable biological substance known to man – and walked up the garden path with a filthy face, stripped down to my jeans. Celia was covered in the same multi-coloured war paint and was, well, just stripped down. We walked slowly towards the house and Mark greeted us at the kitchen door, asked how things had gone and was delighted to hear of the successful outcome. I was pleased that he was delighted and moreso that he didn't seem to notice anything unusual about our appearance. Hubert was indeed a fortunate chap to be able to enjoy magnificent views of the Cotswolds every working day, but I felt it was unlikely that he would ever again enjoy the wonderful views he had seen that day.

Throughout the decade things were slowly, but significantly, changing in the world of farm veterinary practice. Vet practitioners everywhere were aware that there were fewer call-outs to the farms. There were sound economic reasons why this was happening but sad ones all the same. Instead, the small animal, the companion animal side of the practice, was expanding quickly and the response had to be fast to satisfy the demands of the pet-owning public. If a professional vacancy arose in the practice, the job seemed only to attract those vets interested in the welfare of companion animals. Their vision of the future of veterinary practice was probably right, but these youngsters missed out on an awful lot of fun.

So in a short space of time we were assumed by our clients to be experts in the world of small animals. I may inadvertently be giving the impression that we were not already competent in this field. We had to be, the Royal College kept an eye on that. There were still days devoted to the TB testing of cattle but that day probably began and ended with small animal surgeries, and in between the cat and dog emergencies were somehow fitted in – all without the aid of the now obligatory mobile phone.

What we were lacking was the veterinary specialist, the person whom today the general practising vet is able to contact at any time for advice or an urgent second opinion. Beyond the Vet Schools there was really nobody to turn to when you were unsure of how to deal with a particular problem. The university specialist was more than willing to see your patient, and although they were often overwhelmed with requests from local practitioners, their advice and support was extremely useful. Following a lengthy telephone conversation and surgical instructions, the consultant often ended the viva with, 'It's really not that difficult, have a shot at it yourself.'

'I might need to think about it.'

'Okay. Let me know how you get on. Good luck.' The upshot of this was, of course, that we were forced into performing operations that initially we would have preferred to refer.

Prime examples of this situation – and there were scores of them – were the dogs with a rupture of their cruciate ligaments. The condition obviously existed when we were at Vet School, but there was no emphasis attached to it and we were not taught how to correct it. Strangely it seemed to be a rare condition in the human field at that time. Forty years on and the reverse seems true: the stars of the rugby and football world are hobbling into their doctors' surgeries and the dogs are lined up at the vets with the same complaint.

It was time for reluctant action when George, a mature black Labrador, hobbled into my surgery one day. I discussed my diagnosis with his young lady owner, who happened to work in the orthopaedic department at the Cheltenham hospital. The abnormal movements of one of his stifle joints cried out for surgical exploration and a probable repair of his ruptured ligaments. George had great difficulty standing and needed help without too much delay. Analgesics would minimise the pain but he needed an operation now. It might have been possible to fit him in for an operation at the Bristol Vet School in about a month's time. Taking a deep breath I informed the owner of my decision. I would operate the next day. I could hear the words of the Vet School surgeon: 'It's quite straightforward', and 'Let me know how you get on.' Funny how he never asked, 'By the way, is your professional negligence premium paid up to date?'

The following morning, after a sleepless night, it was time to commence the day's operative surgery. George was prepared for surgery in our routine manner. RANA Rosemary took control of the anaesthesia. Surgical assistant Debbie scrubbed up and, at appropriate times, passed me the instruments that I requested. I began the operation. Having surgically explored the joint, it was my intention to replace the ruptured anterior (now referred to as the cranial), ligament with a prosthesis. My technique of choice was Patsaama's method, where my skin prosthesis would be inserted through femoral and tibial bone tunnels and anchored at either end. I approached the stifle joint from the lateral aspect by a parapatellar skin incision which extended from the lower third of the femur to the upper third of the tibia. I then incised the underlying fascia together with the joint capsule to open the joint. I dislocated the patella medially to expose the trochlea and infrapatellar pad of fat. With Debbie's assistance, I drilled the femoral tunnel from just above the origin of the lateral collateral ligament. The drill emerged on the medial surface of the lateral condyle at the point of attachment of the cranial cruciate ligament. With the stifle joint in maximum flexion I drilled the tibial tunnel from the intercondyloid fossa so that it emerged towards the distal extremity of the tibial crest.

I cut a 4mm skin transplant the length of, and parallel with, the edge of my initial skin incision. I passed the skin through the femoral and tibial tunnels by twisting it up and attaching a length of monofilament wire to one end, and then passed the wire through the femoral tunnel and pulled the skin through. The wire then continued down through the tibial tunnel, followed by the skin prosthesis. I repositioned the patella in the trochlea. I anchored the skin transplant at the femoral tunnel by suturing it to the joint capsule and fascia with two mattress sutures of monofilament nylon and cut off the excess skin. I extended the stifle and pulled the skin transplant tight, reflecting its end over the tibial crest, and attached it to the fascia with another two mattress sutures of the monofilament. I co-apted the joint capsule and fascia with mattress sutures and closed the skin incision with interrupted sutures of monofilament nylon. I then washed my hands and had a cup of strong tea.

While George recovered from his anaesthetic Rosemary applied a Robert-Jones dressing; a heavily padded cotton wool bandage from one end of his leg to the other.

In his hospital kennel George gradually and quietly recovered during the day and awaited the arrival of his owner. Naturally, after the initial 'How is he?', she asked the next inevitable question: 'How did the operation go?'

'Very well', Debbie replied.

'Were there any complications?' she queried.

'None at all; everything went perfectly', replied my young, inexperienced and too-truthful-for-her-own-good nurse.

'Has Mr Smith done many of these operations?' That was definitely the wrong question to ask honest Debbie.

'He hasn't actually done this particular operation before so he had his surgery book open on the operating table all the time telling him how to do it.'

Debbie survived many years in our practice without me ever getting round to gagging her. When she left our practice we lost an excellent nurse. Sadly, I believe her admirable qualities became ignored and unappreciated by a 'paper qualifications only' workplace society, and more than three decades later the same argument as to whether the veterinary profession should recognise experienced 'unqualified' nurses rumbles on. I suspect her reasons were a combination of knowing that without formal paper qualifications she would be unable to rise to the position of Head Nurse, which I think she undoubtedly deserved, but also feeling that she was possibly blocking the career opportunity of a younger qualified person.

George's owner was happy and a few weeks later I knew he was too. He was walking soundly. More than a few thanks were also due to the surgical textbook notes of my university mentors. Some things in life you have to do by the book. To reassure any concerned owners who may be reading this, I managed to complete the third operation without reference to any book. Today I could almost carry out the procedure in my sleep. I much prefer to dream of other things these days. Despite all this justification for DIY surgery, unless the animal's treatment was an emergency, it was usually of enormous benefit to make an appointment with a consultant member of staff at our nearby Bristol Vet School even if it meant a wait of a week or two.

One mysterious case involved a Springer Spaniel called Rufus. His owner was an officer at RAF Innsworth. When his dog began to vomit occasionally, I was not too concerned because dogs are opportunist eaters and the dog that has never been sick from ingestion of rubbish of some description has probably never existed. I began to get more concerned when he failed to respond to increasingly sophisticated treatments. His abdomen did not feel especially abnormal when I palpated it and I certainly could not feel anything resembling a hard foreign body. I gave Rufus a general anaesthetic and X-rayed his abdomen. There was nothing particularly abnormal to be seen on the radiographs to account for his problem and yet I had an intuitive feeling that the stomach was not as it should be. More X-rays – following barium swallows to outline any abnormalities – still did not convince me that there was justification for carrying out an exploratory laparotomy and taking a look inside his stomach.

A trip to Bristol University would allow an examination of his stomach with an endoscope. In due course, after yet more X-rays had been taken, the surgeon carried out the endoscopy examination. Within minutes the investigative tip of the instrument brushed against something strange. There was indeed a gastric foreign body present: the surgeon had discovered a piece of clothing. He clamped on to it with the tiny grasping jaws of his endoscope and slowly withdrew the small garment. I can only guess what he said when he pulled it out through the dog's mouth. We chatted over the telephone and, later that day, I rang the owners to give them the news of Rufus' successful visit to the Vet School. His owner's wife's response to my good news was a bit surprising.

'Look, I do believe you, Mr Smith, when you say they found a bikini top in our dog's stomach, but the thing that concerns me most is that neither I nor my daughter has ever owned a mauve bikini.'

It was unfortunate that a newspaper reporter lived close by. The next day both the local and national newspapers were urgently seeking the owner of the bottom half of a mauve bikini.

CHAPTER SEVEN

WHEN THE PHYLLOSAN
STOPS WORKING

Friendly gossip is a normal part of village life and I always enjoyed chatting to friends and neighbours I met in the street. Invariably the conversation turned to animals but it was good to feel that you were part of the community. Naturally, you sometimes talked about the pets' owners too, but a strange event occurred at the beginning of the 1980s that got the villagers gossiping about *me*.

To set the scene I must tell you about a wonderful Irishman who often brought his animals to our surgery. He lived in Somerford Keynes, not far from Cirencester, but on his daily journey to work he passed through Churchdown on his way to Staverton Airport. His name was John F. McDonnell, but his friends knew him as Mac. During the war years he had piloted planes for the RAF but now he flew his planes commercially, and one of his clients was Ordnance Survey, the map makers. It was always fascinating to hear him relating his wartime stories — with his humorous anecdotes he could easily have written *'Allo 'Allo*.

I cannot remember how he learned of my interest in fishing, but once he had, every time we met he would invite me out to fish the lake at his country home. Stupidly, I was always too busy to accept his kind invitation until one day, when a very subdued Mac came into surgery with his Border Collie for treatment. I had very recently put his German Shepherd to sleep following a visit to the Bristol Vet School, where it was confirmed that he was suffering from a cancerous illness for which there was no successful treatment. Tragically, Mac told me that his wife, Doreen, had also died in the last week from a cancer-related illness. He seemed so alone that when he mentioned fishing I felt obliged to accept his invitation.

The next free Saturday, son Ed, who was twelve at the time, and I zoomed off in our little red MG, armed with just a couple of fishing rods. We pulled into the gravel parking area in front of the large bungalow, where Mac was waiting to welcome us to Willow Pool. He escorted us through to his lounge, and, through the large patio windows, I cast my eyes for the first time upon the beautiful lake at the rear of the house. As a bonus there were two other lakes begging to be fished. I'll refrain from further angling talk except to say that by the end of that afternoon we had landed a pike that weighed in excess of 20lb (and whose enormous jaws grabbed a simple famous lure, a Shakespeare 'Little S' plug), and cemented a warm Anglo-Irish friendship that would last for twenty years. Sadly, Mac died in 2005; by then we had come to look on him as one of the family.

We were keen to fit into village life, however, shortly after our arrival, we found ourselves making front page news.

It was not unusual for passing motorists to leave an injured animal on our doorstep, and it was often the early morning worker who was the first to encounter the unlucky creature that had come to grief with a speeding car in the night. Thus, when our postman, Colin Payne, arrived with our veterinary mail early one cold January morning he assumed a blanketed parcel left by the front door was just such an animal – he was therefore amazed to hear the cry of a newborn baby coming from the parcel.

That morning I was aware of Angela calling upstairs at about 7.45 as she left to drive the children to school. 'We're off now' she shouted up, and, almost as an afterthought, 'Someone has left a poor old accident cat on the doorstep for you to look after'. 'Okay' I mumbled into my pillow as I drifted back into a wonderful dream involving fishing.

I knew my wife was back when, an hour later, she yelled up the stairs, 'Ive, you have to get up now!' There was an unusual urgency in her voice.

'Okay, I'm coming.'

'Ive, there are police and detectives all over the place.'

'What? Why?'

'Because it wasn't a cat on the doorstep.'

'What was it then?'

'It was a baby!'

On discovery, Colin had taken the baby to the house next door where our neighbour, Viv Hawkes, nursed the baby – a little girl – until the ambulance arrived and rushed her to the maternity unit in Gloucester. It did not take long for the nurses there to give her a name, and 'Joy' was soon recovering from her ordeal.

By 1 p.m. the story was a major item on the BBC news. On arrival at the surery, I found it rather amusing to watch the pushing and jostling of two rival television crews keen to interview me and was thoroughly enjoying my fifteen minutes of fame until I realised why they were interested in me – they suspected that I was the father!

'No, this has never actually happened here before.' I replied to an eager journalist. (I felt like saying, 'Well, only every other Thursday'.)

'How old is your wife Mr Smith?' That appeared to be a very important question.

'Thirty-one going on thirty-two', I replied. Well, she didn't look any older.

'Have you any idea why the baby was left on *your* doorstep?' The questions were becoming increasingly personal.

'None at all, pal', I replied.

'Have you any idea who the mother might be?'

'None at all.' I could sense their disappointment.

The questioning continued at intervals throughout the day and by 3 p.m. I'd had enough. The ITV reporter dropped a clapperboard, asked me another personal question, before finally realising I'd had a bad day and leaving.

As chance would have it, the monthly meeting of the Cotswold Veterinary Society was held that evening at the Cleeveway Hotel in Bishops Cleeve. By then it had become abundantly clear why everyone was so interested in me. I knew that I would have to run the gauntlet in the hotel's restaurant confronted by most of my veterinary colleagues. The attendance of meetings at this venue was always excellent. Even if the speaker was rubbish, the buffet, armchairs, and the roaring log fire on a cold night were attractions not to be missed. On arrival, I found it more difficult than usual to find a parking space. For whatever reason there was a particularly full house tonight.

My considerate and ever-supportive professional colleagues behaved in the respectful manner I should have anticipated from them. I had hardly put my foot in the door when a local Irish vet shouted, 'Evening, Ivor. Was it a nurse or one of the receptionists then?'

It had been a stressful few days and I looked forward to a few hours fishing at Willow Pool. Naturally I would have to face Mac's humorous comments on my arrival but he was not to have the opportunity he had anticipated. During my journey to Somerford Keynes a young woman collapsed in Debenhams department store in Gloucester. She was cared for by the manageress and, after explaining that she was the missing mother, she was soon reunited with her baby daughter. By the time I arrived, Mac had heard the radio announcement of this news, but as you can imagine he was still determined to give his wonderful Irish comments on the week's saga. At the end of that day, and a few pike later, I was ready for another week.

Not unexpectedly the surgery was the source of many of our children's pets. They had begged for a cat and I had promised that they could have one from the next litter of unwanted kittens brought to the surgery 'to be disposed of'. Litters of healthy kittens were never put to sleep and, not surprisingly, a litter appeared at surgery shortly before Christmas one year. They had received the usual nursing care and the chubby creatures were ready for new homes. I took Ed and Sally to the surgery and they chose Holly, a pretty tabby female that soon made it clear she wanted no affection from anyone. Within days there was not one hand in the family that did not bear her claw marks. The children were terrified of her and the Christmas morning catastrophe was the last straw.

The morning had been a quiet one and Sally was doing her best to befriend Holly. A few friends had called in for a seasonal drink and chat, asked to see the latest addition to our family, and left with at least one good scratch for their interest. Angela was waist-deep in the cooking and preparation of the Christmas dinner when Dr Jimmy Caldwell, our local GP, called in for a glass of special malt and to wish us well. We needed it. He could have treated us all for cat-bite injuries.

Jimmy was standing next to the Christmas tree when Holly decided to take off. She leapt from Sally's lap and made a bee-line for him. He hadn't time to object to Holly's unwelcome approaches as she climbed his suit trousers and, in a flash, was on his shoulder. He defended himself as the cat clawed at his head before it dived onto the Christmas tree. It became top-heavy and collapsed across the floor of the lounge. Pine needles, broken decorations and fused lights were everywhere. The cat appeared from the midst of the debris like the star of a Walt Disney cartoon. This was a commotion Angela declared she could do without on Christmas day morning. I fully understood her concerns.

Dr Caldwell left shortly after and so too did Holly. We all felt that she would be happier back with her siblings in the surgery. No doubt I should have heeded the advice of the animal societies and not taken on a new pet at Christmas-time. The scratching and biting could have been delayed until the New Year.

The children were told that they could select another kitten the following week. By then another litter had been brought to the surgery 'to be dealt with'. They chose Fluffy, a black and white female who appeared to be a little more placid. Later that week, I was a little perturbed and embarrassed to learn that Holly had been chosen to go to a new home. I didn't have the opportunity to fully warn the new owners that the little cat could be a bit of a handful. In our experience it was often a bleeding handful, and clearly she belonged to a litter of partly feral kittens. I cannot remember where Holly went, but if I was starting a search I would look for a house where no mouse, rat, dog or indeed visitors of any description set foot on the premises.

Out of the frying pan into the fire. That's how it seemed with our children's pets at the time. The new kitten, Fluffy, was placid, cuddly and quiet – a little too quiet. I had checked the health of the litter when they were left with us at the surgery and found no signs of a current infection. But clearly there was. Within days Fluffy developed an illness and was reluctant to drink, feed or play, and she started to sneeze. She was infected with one of the cat flu viruses, feline calicivirus, and numerous painful areas of her mouth and tongue soon became ulcerated. We were feeding her from a syringe just days later. Our efforts to save this patient had not gone unobserved. Dear old Ginny, the mum of two wonderful Labrador litters, had decided to give a helping hand. Astonishingly, within days she had come into milk. For whatever reason, Fluffy did not argue and she had the whole milk bar to herself. She suckled herself into contented sleep.

The daily dose of antibiotics no doubt helped, but Fluffy's survival was in no small measure due to Ginny's maternal instincts. It was a fascinating experience to watch and of course there could not have been stronger bonding behaviour between the two animals.

Ginny was a tremendous pal and had been part of the family for fifteen years. Nevertheless, the old dear was ageing, losing weight and, because of her arthritic joints, found getting around difficult. I kept a close eye on her and I knew that, as so often happens, a tumour like those I had felt a hundred times before in elderly cats and dogs was developing in her liver. Her weight loss eventually became rapid and her weakness suddenly profound, but she still waited at the front door to jump into the car whenever there was any suggestion that I was going fishing. Early one Saturday morning she had recognised the usual sounds of the filling of the thermos flask and the sandwich box lid and was determined not to be left behind. I lifted her into the MG at Churchdown and out of the car on arrival at Mac's. I cannot remember whether I caught any fish that day. I do recall, however, that Ginny made an enormous effort to trot around the lakes as if it were just a normal weekend. I knew that it would be anything but that.

I made it easy for her to pinch a couple of my ham, cheese and Branston Pickle sandwiches. When she looked up at me, questioning whether it was okay to do more than simply examine them on the grass, I spoke no words of objection and she gulped them down. A piece of cake followed. We had a wonderful last day together in the countryside we both loved. Ginny was unable to get back on to her feet after that happy day. Two days later Angela and I sat on the carpet with her in the back room of our home. It was the end of the road for Ginny, this beautiful dog who had given us so much love and pleasure in our lives.

How many times have I heard this expressed from other owners on this emotional occasion? Suddenly we were no different from the owners of the hundreds of pets I had put to sleep. The three of us sat on the carpet in silence. Knowing that within a very short time we would no longer enjoy her being with us was heartbreaking. I don't know what triggered the precise time but at some poignant moment I simply looked at Angela and in the simplest possible way we agreed, 'Okay?' She raised the vein, I injected the painless barbiturate, and Ginny went to sleep for ever. The children arrived home from school later that afternoon. The events of the day had been discussed with them and they accepted the sad task, knowing that they would not be present.

Carrying out euthanasia of any animal is never easy, and always worse when children are present. Naturally I have always felt obliged to respect the owners' wishes, but I nevertheless tried to persuade them that it was really not a good idea for their children to be there. On one occasion the owners of an elderly Collie dog insisted that putting to sleep their faithful old friend must be a family affair, and brought their two young children along to the surgery to say goodbye. As is often the case, many couples bring a four-legged friend ino their family before a two-legged baby arrives – the consequence being that the children grow up not knowing a time when Rover, Felix or Bugsy was not a part of the family. Thus when old Collie Rover had been lifted on to my table, the nurse had clipped and spirited his arm and I approached calmly with a syringe, it was all too much for them. The distressed parents were weeping uncontrollably and the two children were hopelessly bemused by the situation. The young boy suddenly developed a protective role and his shouts to his father, 'Don't let him do it, Dad, don't let him do it!' as he bravely attempted to stop me giving that final injection, still ring in my ears today.

Usually I could professionally switch off from these grief-stricken occasions and for those necessary few minutes just do my job, but it was hard not to let Ginny's death affect me. Perhaps our children were aware of the effect the last few days had had on us, or perhaps they were simply trying to cheer us up when, later that week, they asked:

'Can we have another puppy, Dad?'

'Can we have a kitten?'

'Dad, can we have a puppy *and* a kitten?'

Our unhappiness continued as we watched Ginny's old feline pal, Fluffy, responding to the loss. For many days she explored every part of the house and garden – we often found her in cupboards and other unusual places – searching for her lost 'mum'.

It had been thirty years since I had experienced the heartbreak of losing my first dog. It was on a wintry afternoon in 1953 – when my family lived in Kingsholm Square – that our Gloucester vet, Alasdair Macleod, had called to examine our elderly Collie, Nellie. By chance, that day, 20 November, also happened to be my thirteenth birthday when he put her to sleep.

Despite the setbacks and disappointments that every family suffers, life has to carry on. The decade was off to a demanding start. With a little share of good fortune, things would get much better. Nevertheless, as time goes by you start to accept that you aren't quite the same person that you used to be. The Phyllosan tablets may well give a boost to the over-forties but you begin to appreciate that it will not be too long before you reach fifty! Gradually, you begin to realise that the discomfort you experienced in your back this week will still be there next week.

Picking up the feet to examine a lame horse was no longer a pleasurable challenge and, as time went by, it started to become a problem. I started to fear the call-out to such horses. I knew that if I was really honest with myself, I probably could not do the job properly, not to my own satisfaction anyway. The back problems had started a few years before, following a routine calving at Churchdown's Green Farm.

Farmer John Halford had telephoned early one afternoon to say that one of his cows was having a bit of trouble calving. 'I think she just needs a bit of 'elp', was John's philosophical way of describing things. There seemed to be ample time to do the job and get back for the start of the evening surgery. At the time a young veterinary student was spending time with us gaining practical experience and learning all the things that they don't teach you at college. He was eager to learn, and I was keen to inspire him. We bundled all the equipment we might need into the back of the car and were at the farm in minutes. In customary fashion Farmer John had provided the obligatory bucket of hot water, soap and towel, and soon the recumbent patient was prepared for her obstetrical examination. I was anxious for things to go smoothly and quickly, firstly to be back in surgery in good time, and secondly to impress our student of my competence and obstetrical skills. In hindsight it was a recipe for disaster.

Within minutes I realised this was not going to be my day. In the depths of her uterus the cow's predicament was instantly apparent. Without describing the situation in technical terms, the oversized calf's head was pointing in one direction and its four legs and tail were pointed in another. There was very little room to manoeuvre the calf into a delivery position but an exhausting hour later the front legs and the head were all pointing the right way. It had been an hour of veterinary masochism but I was chuffed at the result and hoped the student was duly impressed. I was clapped out, but I tried to act as if it was all just in a day's work. John and the student hauled on the ropes attached to the head and legs and another calf slid into our world.

Diane, John's wife, produced a welcome tray of tea and biscuits and as we supped and chatted I began to load the soiled equipment into the car. I had spent an hour doing a gym routine inside my patient and so lifting things into the car should have been no problem. I had given the tired cow a large beneficial injection of intravenous calcium fluids and I shall never forget reaching forward in the car with the empty bottle. There was a twinge in my lower back, spasm in my lumbar muscles and a sudden excruciating pain that every true back sufferer will have experienced at some time. I tried to shrug it off, without realising that for me it was the start of an ongoing problem.

I somehow managed to drive us back, hobbled into surgery and began the evening session of consultations, pretending that all was well. Two hours or so later, I was for once pleased to see the end of the day and be home enjoying another cup of tea with a large dose of aspirin.

One evening, as I sat reading the *Citizen*, I answered the telephone to Mark Hicks-Beach of Witcombe Park Estates. I expected him to apologise for disturbing me at night as he normally did and then to ask if I would mind going out to look at an animal that he was not happy with. I was therefore greatly surprised when he asked me if I would be interested in doing a parachute jump. Without hesitating I told him I would love to do it, before giving any thought to the implications of what I had just agreed to do. I was, of course, now on the wrong side of forty, but only just. It was to be a charity event and it would take place one Sunday morning over Staverton Airport, on the edge of Cheltenham. I believe that in order to participate in the jump, being under the age of forty was a condition, which meant that the rules were bent or, at the very least, a number of lies were told.

The rules also stated that it was compulsory to have a minimum of six hours of tuition before parachuting. There were about forty volunteer jumpers in all, and the money we raised was to be distributed to Tewkesbury Hospital and other local good causes. My clients responded generously to my request for sponsorship and the sponsor forms on the waiting room noticeboard were filled rapidly. There was no opportunity to back out now. The large sums of money promised spurred me on and I hoped that every one of my sponsors wished me a safe landing. We were in good hands; our instructors were the Parachute Regiment and, as the team's captain stated on many occasions, the only time you can get injured parachuting is when you land on the ground.

I took his words of wisdom and the preparation seriously. Surprisingly, until the day before the jump we had no training at all. The Paras must have had more confidence in us than we had in ourselves. We met up early one Saturday morning at Brockworth School to be instructed in the techniques of leaving the aircraft and controlling the canopy (the proper name for the parachute), and the all-important art of landing. Our six hours of instruction were packed into one day and the afternoon was spent in the school's gym jumping off wooden horses on to a padded mat, landing flat-footed and feet together before pitching into the parachute roll. I had seen the roll done so many times at the cinema it was difficult to understand why it did not come naturally.

I retired to bed that evening with a thumping headache, slept for about two and a half hours and was ready to get up at four o'clock the following morning. I skipped breakfast and was raring to go by seven. I reported for duty at Staverton Airport and fell in. We were lined up and had our photographs taken. I turned to Keith Bawden, my fellow-jumper, and whispered, 'I hope these are not for identification purposes.' We had been divided into groups of eight. I was a member of Drop No. 1 group and we were instructed to board the plane. The weather was awful that Sunday morning and I could not recall having been given instructions on how to control the parachute during adverse conditions.

Paul Quarry was another of my companion jumpers. His questioning observations were apt but a little too late for anything that could influence our destiny.

'They didn't tell us what to do in the middle of a chucking gale, did they?' he commented. At least that's what I think he said, but it was difficult to be sure above the howling wind. It was the first time I had met Paul, but it would not be the last. There were to be many more amusing events ahead of us, and not all of them on English soil. There would be momentous occasions from Dublin to Rome via Paris when we would be patriotic supporters of England Rugby and could say in the future, 'We were there.'

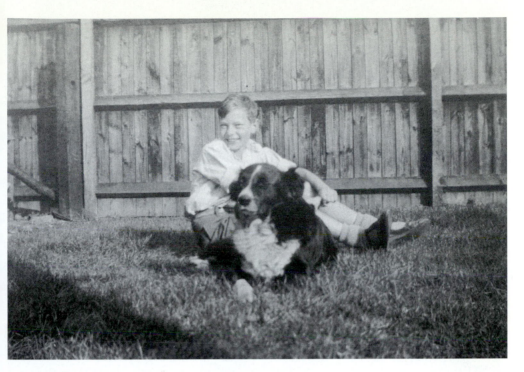

With my first best friend, Nellie, at home in Gloucester, 1950.

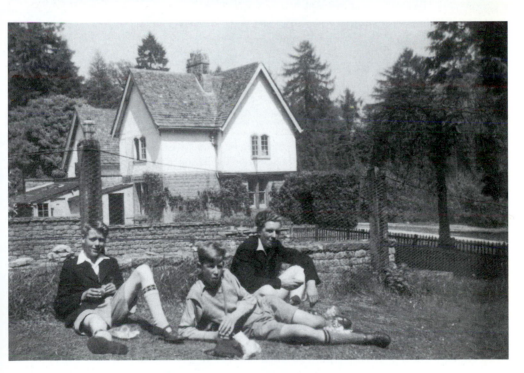

Classmates at Chedworth Roman Villa, 1955. From left to right: Keith Russell, Ted Rudge and Phil Richardson reserving their energy for the long bike ride back to Gloucester.

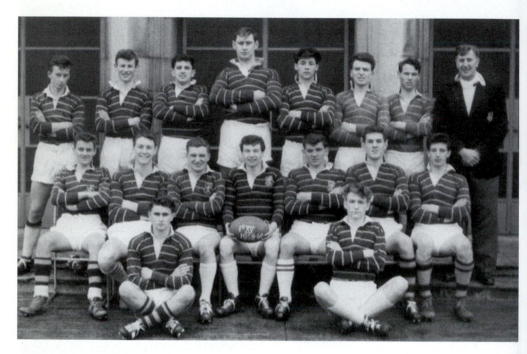

Crypt School 1st XV, 1959/60. Back row: G. Middleton, R. Jones, J. McGarr, P. Hendy, D. Powell, R. Eggleton, C. Richards, Mr H.O. Edwards. Middle row: D. Johnson, E. Newton, P. Richardson, I. Smith, R. Hannaford, M. Pickard, D. Simmons. Front row: G. Dalby, C. Grafton.

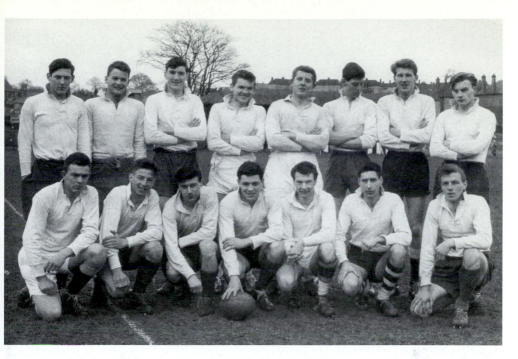

Gloucestershire Schools Rugby XV, 1959, captained by Trevor Wintle, who would shortly become England's number one scrum-half. I'm in the front row, third from the right.

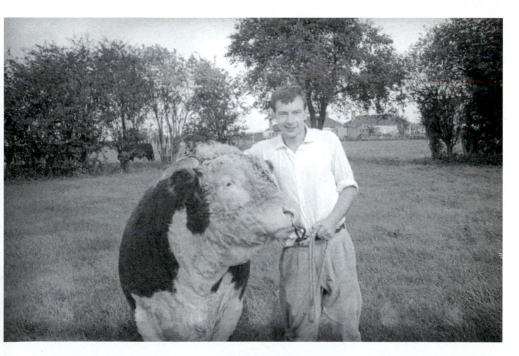

Getting to know the bulls, 1961. Vacation work at the MMB artificial insemination centre at Longford.

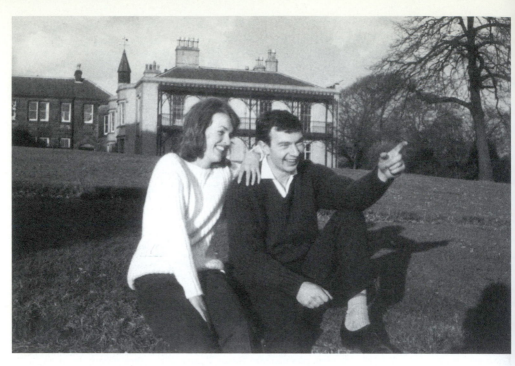

An occasional visitor to Greenbank, an annexe of Derby Hall's hall of residence, 1961. Angela was sneaked into neighbouring Dale Hall at night, the ladies' student residence.

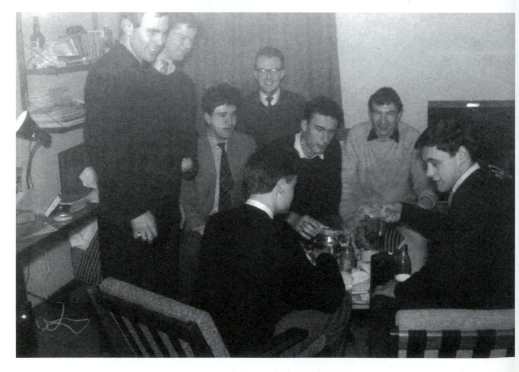

Late night beverages at Derby Hall, 1962. Half of this lot were insomniac students from our year at the Faculty of Veterinary Science.

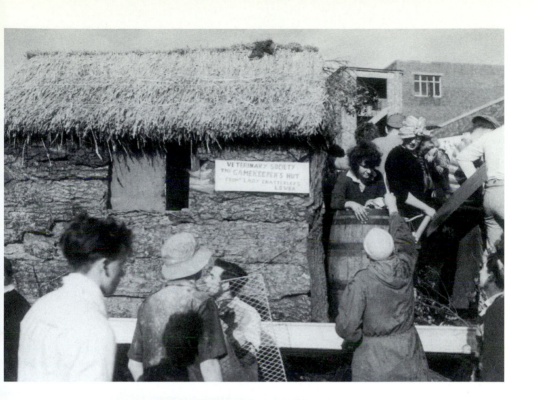

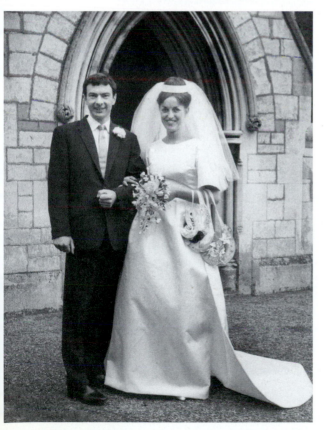

Above: Liverpool University students' charity panto procession, 1961.

Left: Wedding bells at Hucclecote, 1963. Ivor and Angela are married at St Philip and St James's Church.

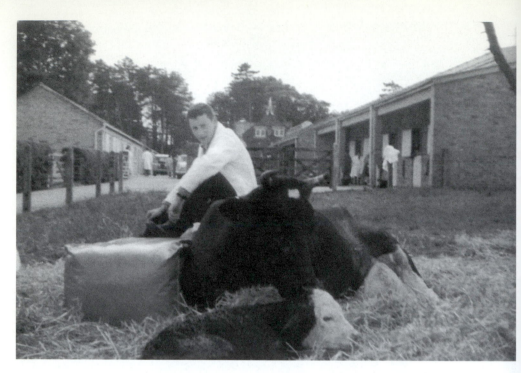

Nigel in charge of the post-operative recovery of a bovine Caesar at Leahurst, 1965.

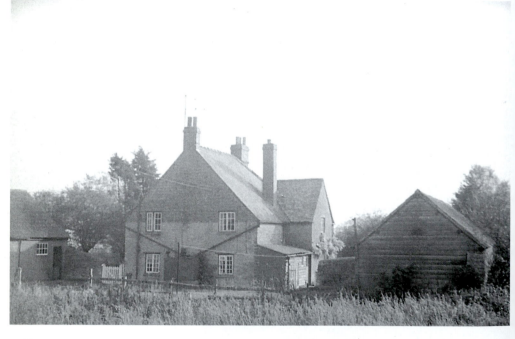

Odd Farm, Crudwell, 1966. Our first rural home – mice and all!

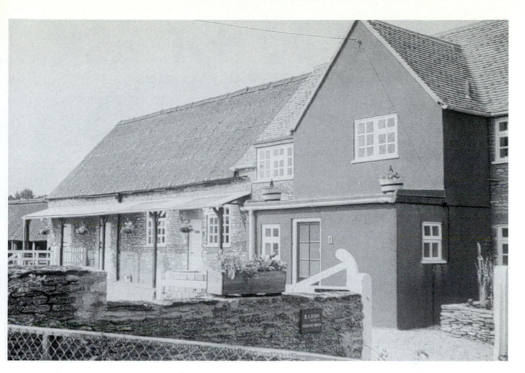

Ridgeway Veterinary Hospital, Crudwell – complete with hanging baskets – in 1967.

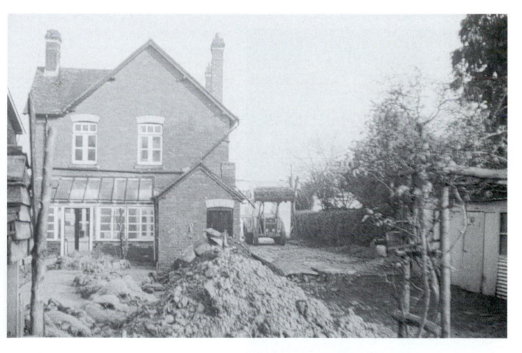

The Churchdown practice, 1972. Week one and the builders start work on the surgery.

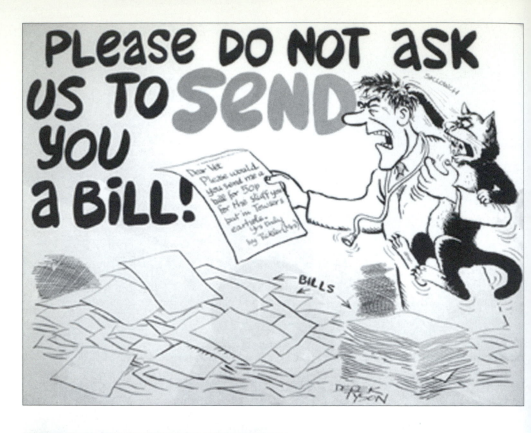

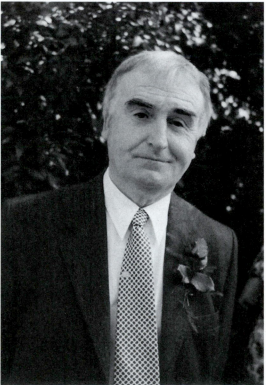

Above: Getting to grips with running my own business in the '70s, as depicted by Gloucester cartoonist Derek Tyson.

Left: A true friend: John Eggleton (1941–2000), pictured here in 1992.

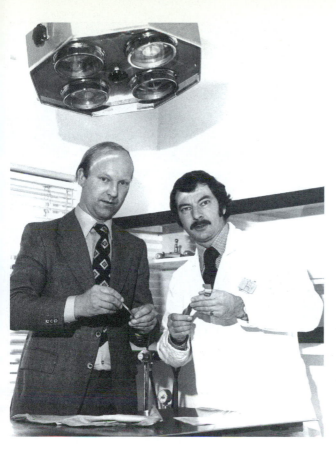

Left: As a veterinary representative of Arnolds, the specialist surgical instrument company, John Troth was a regular visitor to the surgery. He is seen here on the left in 1976.

Below: Her Majesty's Silver Jubilee celebrations, 1977. Farmer Ben Pullen heading a trailer full of youngsters passes the veterinary surgery in Albemarle Road.

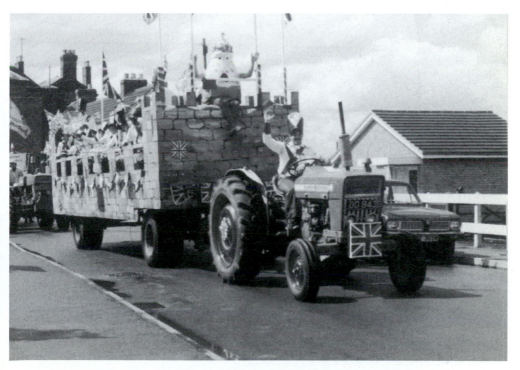

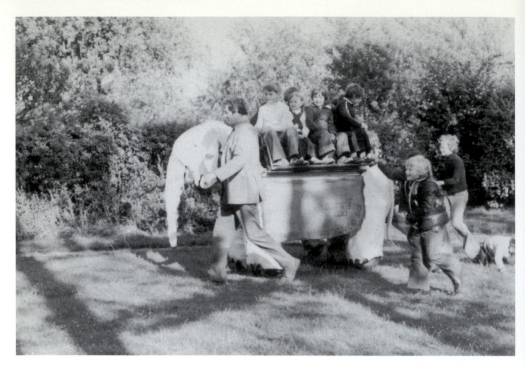

There were countless rides after the procession when Uncle Adam Pullen entertained walking the elephant.

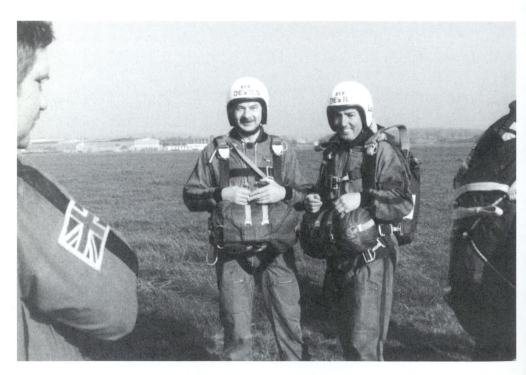

The Red Devils Air Display (Extra B) Team, 1981. Ivor and Mark Hicks-Beach prepared for the jump of their lives.

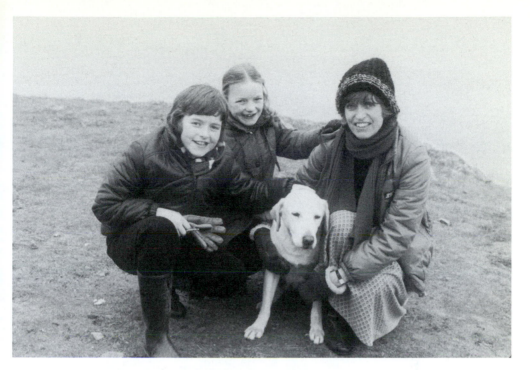

A few hours break with the family at the top of the Malverns, 1982. From left to right: Ed, Sally, Labrador Ginny, and Angela.

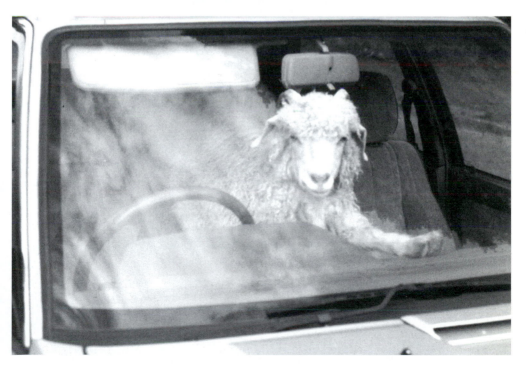

Clients generally wait patiently at the surgery, some in the waiting room, some in their cars. This well-behaved goat was chauffeured to surgery from Coopers Hill Farm by Miss Metson.

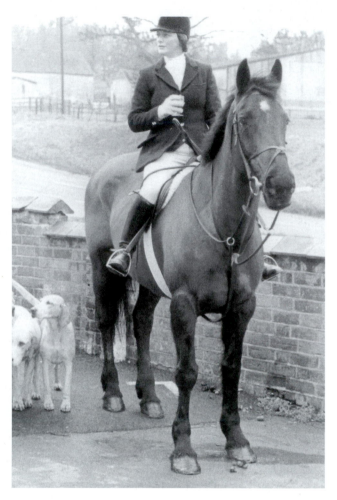

Judy Pullen riding post-operative mare Moffet, 1979. Moffet
recovered from her injuries – seen here with deep chest scars
under the breast plate – and went on to have a colt foal,
Soup Dragon, who competed at Burghley, Badminton, and at
international level.

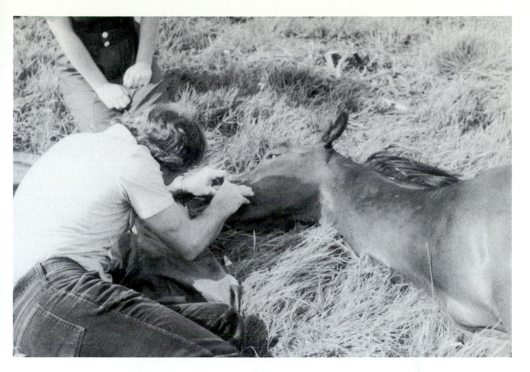

Dental surgery under field conditions in 1981 – and still using Immobilon.

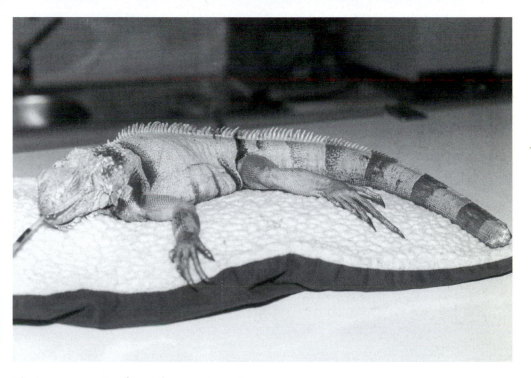

The iguana recovering from tail surgery in 1996.

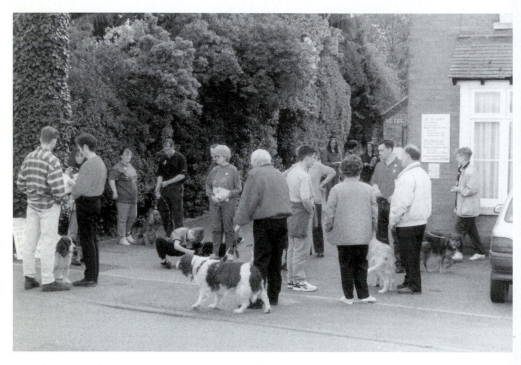

National Pets' Week, 1995. The dogs, their owners and The Brambles' staff gather at the surgery in Churchdown for the start of a charity walk over Chosen Hill.

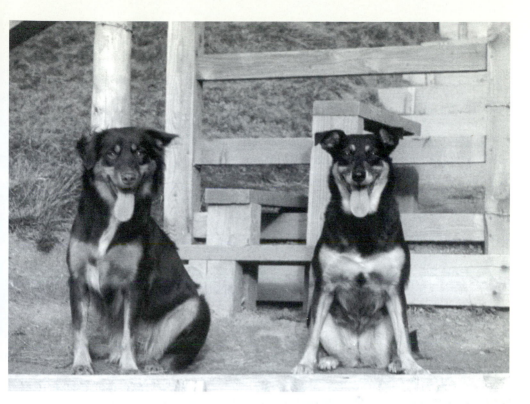

A youthful Coco (left) with her mum, Jimmy, on an early morning run over Chosen Hill, 1991.

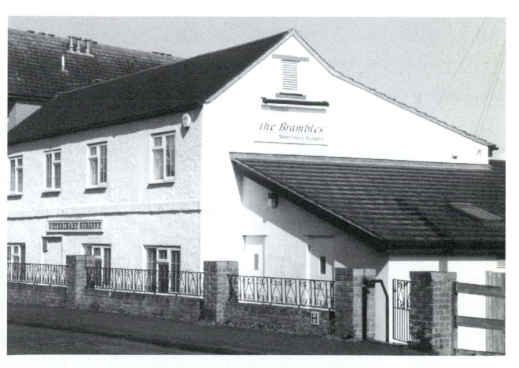

The Brambles veterinary surgery in 2008.

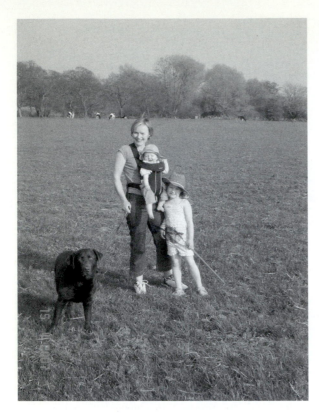

Left: Daughter Sally with granddaughters Darcey and Millie in rural Derbyshire in 2007 – and not forgetting Bramble, of course.

Below: Ivor and Bramble enjoying retired life on the River Ecclesbourne, 2008.

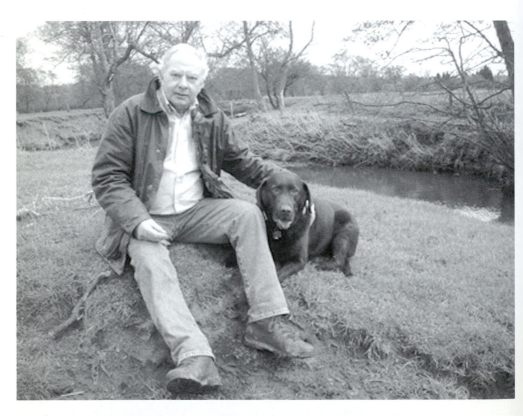

As the plane flew higher I could not help thinking to myself, 'Don't you get yourself into some silly situations Ivor?' But this was something I had always wanted to do. I had seen many war films and had always wondered how the chaps must have felt jumping out of a plane. I was soon to find out. Thank heavens we did not have to worry about somebody shooting at us on the way down. Mark Hicks-Beach was to be first out. He was ordered to move to the exit point. The plane flew over the target area, a large cross unmistakably marked out on the fields below us. He was told to jump. He didn't exactly refuse, but he gave the burly Para sergeant the impression that he would like a bit more time to think about it. The plane circled a second time and when it reached the drop zone again Mark was given some extra encouragement from the sergeant's helping hand.

As my turn approached I was aware of my heart rate and blood pressure rising. 'Now's your time to discover what it *does* feel like to jump out of a plane', I thought to myself for the final time. The sergeant said something I could not hear, but he winked at me and I dived out into the clouds in crucifix fashion the way I had seen John Wayne do it several times in the movies. Once out the instructors stressed that you should look over your shoulder and count – a thousand and one – a thousand and two – a thousand and check. At that point if your canopy had not opened it was advantageous to release the reserve parachute strapped to your body. For some reason as I dived out over the Gloucestershire terrain the counting routine became superfluous.

My spectacular swallow dive, aided by a blast of air from below, became an upside-down dive and I watched with relief as the canopy opened above me. For several minutes I seemed to hang suspended in a silent world as the noise of the plane's engines retreated into the distance. It was a magical experience, but I was aware that I had to do something to improve my chances of surviving the fall. I recalled that if I pulled on the left rope I would go in one direction and if I pulled on the right rope I might go in the other, and that was how I was going to hit the target, which was somewhere in the vicinity of Staverton Airport. I wish they didn't keep referring to the target as a cross on the tarmac. It was a short but very exciting experience, as the little matchboxes and specks on the ground started to look like factory roofs, vehicles and trees. And Lord, was that a motorway or just a dual carriageway over there? I then started to worry about the 'only time you can get hurt' scenario.

It was so gusty it became a mammoth task trying to control the parachute. Within seconds I knew I would be back on *terra firma*, and as the ground rushed up to greet me I knew I had failed to keep both feet together as one ankle complained of the ordeal. As for the parachute roll, the strength of the wind dragging both the parachute and me across the field prevented one of any description being attempted. Better luck next time. But sadly there will not be a next time. There is no doubt how exhilarating this sport is, but it is sensibly left for the youngsters to enjoy.

We were not without our walking wounded on this occasion. Our team leader Mark suffered an ankle fracture and there were more serious injuries. Following our initial Sunday drop a decision was made to postpone further jumps until weather conditions improved. It was a sensible move but there is no doubt in my mind that the rest of that plucky gang of Brits would have done their jump that day regardless of the awful weather. It was a bonding occasion and two fellows who were distant acquaintances to me at the beginning of that day, Keith, an antique furniture restorer, and Paul, a local businessman, became lifelong friends.

Back at home we were still suffering the loss of Ginny. She had always been with us wherever we went, whether it was holidays, shopping, fishing trips or the regular scrambles over Chosen Hill. We were resigned to the fact that we would never have another dog. Nothing could possibly replace her. How many times have I heard this statement from my clients? That individual companion, be it dog, cat, rabbit or gerbil, cannot be replaced. But there is always room for the company of another infuriating, demanding, house disrupting, beloved animal. In our case, for better or for worse, it was to be Jimmy.

I was a bit late for surgery one morning having spent at least twenty minutes on the telephone advising a worried client on the care and management of rearing a one-month-old puppy. Apparently this little dog had reached her via the local rugby club. How this puppy had been passed from pillar to post to her husband is another story, but by 9 o'clock the puppy was at the practice. I walked into the kennel room and asked, 'Who's this little chap?' I was first astounded and then a little amused to find that it was the very same puppy I had been discussing for the last half-hour.

'Well, that was a good way to start the day', I thought to myself. 'Things will no doubt get better.' Many days began like this anyway.

I finished morning surgery and wandered into the animal room to check on the patients relaxing in their kennels, awaiting their moment to be transferred to the operating theatre. I passed along a line of animals until I reached an end kennel where I found the unexpected patient, the abandoned black-and-tan puppy. Already it had been examined by one of the vets, and the nurses had fed and wormed it and given the sort of TLC treatment that they do so much better than me. It was now on four regular feeds a day and would grow rapidly. I dislike referring to people's pets as 'it' but there was a specific reason in this case.

The puppy was with us for a second week and during that time our son, Ed, had begun routinely visiting it after school. When we left the surgery he would turn to the end kennel and call to the pup, 'We'll see you, Jimmy.' At this time, in 1983, one of the most popular comedians of the day was Russ Abbot and the 'Jimmy' reference was one of his catchphrases. By the third weekend with us son Ed's Sunday request was, 'Can we have him at home this afternoon, Dad?' That was the last day Jimmy spent in the surgery. That afternoon was spent on the lawn. The little dog that I had taken scant interest in other than its health and welfare was to become a family member and would be very much part of our life for the next thirteen years. All I had to do now was explain to everyone why our dog was given a boy's name. Jimmy was a girl.

As a result of her poor start she was weak on her legs and walked with difficulty, but she gained weight rapidly and became stronger by the day. At three months old she was a healthy, normal puppy. We had no idea who or what her parents were. She could have been related to just about any of the popular breeds in our area, and probably was. At about a year old I began to suspect that she had inherited mainly the features of a Doberman and a German Shepherd, definitely a Collie, and some Labrador. Out walking, folks were complimentary and often remarked, 'Oh, what a lovely dog, what breed is she?'

Depending on the enquirer I would often reply, 'She's a Gloucester Terrier.' 'Oh really? I haven't seen one of those before' was a frequent response.

Jimmy had much to live up to and she did not let us down. She was a lovable dog, but as a result of her unusual pedigree gave the impression to some that she could be ferocious. For a relatively small dog she was disproportionately strong. Like Ginny before her, she became a regular fishing companion and was a remarkable swimmer. She loved to retrieve sticks thrown into the lake and at times I was quite stunned by the size of fallen branches she would haul around in the hope that they would be thrown for her to bring back.

Unwisely, I never got round to carrying out the operation of spaying her. I strongly recommended the operation to my clients but for some reason, either I never found the time or perhaps because of a subconscious reluctance to operate on my own dog, a hysterectomy was not performed at the appropriate time. The obvious advantages of spaying the young bitch are to avoid unwanted pregnancies and to prevent the development of diseases of the reproductive system in later life. Pyometra is one of the common conditions where the uterus fills with pathological secretions and often develops after the bitch has been in season.

Jimmy had turned eight and had recently been in season when we noticed that she had started to become a little lethargic and uncharacteristically indifferent towards her food. She seemed more interested in her water bowl. The signs of a possible uterine disease were beginning and I felt that the writing was on the wall for surgery in the very near future. Late one evening, when the family had turned in for the night, I found myself sitting in our back room snug watching the television news. Jimmy was curled up in her bed on the opposite side of the room, her head resting on her paws and one eye fixed on me. This was her usual behaviour, watching and anticipating my next move, just in case it was her cue to accompany me on a stroll around our large garden, or a trip in the car on a night-time call-out.

'You don't look very ill to me', I muttered to her. She lay there almost with a glint in her eye. The penny suddenly dropped. 'I don't believe this', I murmured to myself. 'You're not ill, you're flipping pregnant!' I dived towards her and it took less than twenty seconds to confirm my suspicions. Deep in her abdomen I could feel with certainty the developing foetuses, which were at the palpable golf ball stage, an immensely diagnostically rewarding stage when you feel them in the abdomen of someone else's dog.

How could this have happened? Jimmy rarely left our company and definitely had not disappeared recently, even for a few minutes. Clearly, if she had not been out of our garden, some dog had been in (excuse the pun). I felt like a Victorian father about to charge around the village looking for the scoundrel with my blunderbuss, but in this instance with a scalpel in hand. After the initial shock I felt more than a little embarrassed. How was I going to live this one down? The options were to allow her to have the puppies or to carry out a hysterectomy at this late stage. The latter was associated with unnecessary surgical risks, and was over-ruled anyway by the other members of the family.

Unsportingly, Jimmy chose my weekend off duty to go into labour. On the Friday evening she became increasingly restless and it was apparent things were about to happen. First stage labour had commenced and the pups were moving into the correct position for a natural birth, before the second stage commenced and a few good strains would pop the puppies out one by one. I am sure she was intent on going for the first stage labour record. At midnight I injected her with a mild sedative and she pretended to sleep. I accompanied her on the other side of the room and also pretended to sleep. Every fifteen minutes we eyeballed each other.

Angela was up shortly before 6 o'clock. Jimmy, however, seemed unaware that there was an important job to be done. Perhaps she knew that this was our fishing weekend and wanted to cause no unnecessary inconvenience. She had at last started to make more of an effort when Angela asked, 'What are you going to do then?' All thoughts of that day's mighty pike about to engulf my lure disappeared. Jimmy had decided I would not go fishing without her. It was time for serious action. I topped up her sedation and enjoyed my usual working breakfast: two half-pint mugs of tea followed by a half-pint mug of coffee.

At 9 o'clock I gave Jimmy her intravenous anaesthetic and looked into her eyes as it took effect. I am sure that she trusted me implicitly as she fell asleep. It was an odd feeling, but I was reluctant to pass on the job to one of my vet colleagues and once she was prepared for surgery and draped up, it suddenly and strangely once more became just another job to be done. Making the initial abdominal incision was no different from the hundreds of others I had carried out. I continued incising the abdominal muscles, the peritoneum and exposed the uterus and the first protruding glimpse of Jimmy's new family. I incised the body of the uterus and gently squeezed a puppy towards the incision, lifted it from its foetal membranes and said hello to the first of Jimmy's pups. It was a large black and white Collie-type dog and my mind started to wonder about the black and white Romeo collies that wandered around our village. The intriguing part of the operation was quickly over and a further five puppies joined the first. Surgical closure of the uterine incision and the repair of the abdomen were straightforward.

Jimmy's mammary glands were beginning to enlarge and as she came round from the anaesthetic Angela had already introduced a lively litter to the canine milk bar. Four of the puppies were black and white and two were a dark chocolate brown. One of the brown ones was destined to become another close member of our family for a very long time. Naming that puppy was not too difficult; daughter Sally called her Coco. Regardless of the animal species, the caesarean was the operation that always gave me the most enjoyment and satisfaction. Operating on Jimmy was routine surgery once I had started and it was not until I looked at her through the stainless-steel bars of her hospital kennel that I suddenly realised that this was no ordinary patient. But I am sure that every single animal I ever had on the operating table was not an ordinary patient to someone.

This trepidation must have been the feeling my clients experienced as they walked to the surgery entrance along the tarmac drive. Often they would be greeted by the chirping of birds from the large aviary next door. They belonged to our neighbours, Tony and Jacqui Rumney, who had bravely moved into their house in the '80s. It must take courage to live next door to a veterinary surgery, but they admit the experience often provided them with some unexpected entertainment. It was common practice for farmers to bring calves, sheep and occasionally goats to the surgery in trailers and horseboxes where they were examined and treated. Ewes that were experiencing lambing difficulties were dealt with on the drive and, if necessary, a caesarean operation was carried out with the patient resting on straw bales. I would have thought that this was enough drama for any family, but obviously this was not the case.

Jacqui's son, Lyndon Davies, was for many years involved in the acting profession. His opportunity arose when pupils from Churchdown's

Chosen Hill School were auditioned for a major role in Dennis Potter's *The Singing Detective*. Knowing him so well, it came as no surprise to learn that he had been successful. Once, while enjoying a glass of coke at our house, I asked him casually what sort of day he'd had. Twelve-year-old Lyndon stroked his brow and replied, 'Oh, not so good, Ivor, I've been through purgatory today.' I cannot recall what the dramatic comment referred to, but he must have been having a bad day.

Little did we know that within a very short time we would be enjoying his Shakespearean roles on stage at the Globe and at Stratford-upon-Avon. While next door one day, I was more than a little surprised when, nearest to the ringing telephone, Tony asked me to answer it and on the other end of the line Dame Judi Dench asked to speak to Lyndon!

At our house one day Angela rushed to the front door to greet Lyndon, knowing that he had secured another successful role. She opened the door, hugged him, and, before she had the chance to wish him the traditional actor's 'break a leg', they tumbled over and Angela fractured an ankle-bone. Lyndon, as young Perkins, appeared regularly in *Sharpe's Rifles* but the opportunity to go to our local for a pint with Sean Bean sadly did not arise.

Jimmy and her family had taken over both the utility room and the kitchen of our house. We still have the treasured video of the litter that Tony took when the pups were a month old – bounding around the house while their proud mum does her best to keep them in line. How different they were from Jimmy at that age. No excuses, but my tardy surgical oversight resulted in years of happiness for five other families, and incalculable happy memories for ours. Coco stayed with us for the next thirteen years.

This episode in our lives took up many fascinating hours but I was also responsible for the health and welfare of hundreds of other clients' four-legged friends. The companion animal side of the practice was growing rapidly, but, disappointingly and frustratingly, the farm side of the practice, in keeping with the national trend, was gradually contracting. In the mid-1980s, probably 40 per cent of practice work revolved around life on the farm. There were still scores of milk-producing farms within a 15-mile radius of Churchdown, and I also spent at least one day of the week involved in the maintenance of the health of numerous large pig farms in the Cotswold area.

Today, most of those pig farms have disappeared and the dairy farms in the area have reduced to a mere handful. The lack of support that successive governments have given to the farming community has, in my view, been little short of scandalous, but this is not the time to debate politics. Fortunately for my practice the loss of income from agriculture was balanced by the increased number of people bringing their pets to the surgery. Many of our clients lived in the Brockworth and Hucclecote areas of Gloucester and, due to lack of public transport at the time, and in many cases no transport at all, demanded a local surgery. So, in 1983, I bought our second surgery. It was a seventeenth-century cottage and adjacent outbuildings in Green Street which, long ago, had once been Brockworth's village blacksmith: hence it was appropriate to name the surgery the Old Forge. In creating an up-to-date and hygeinic surgery, I had hoped to retain most of the original building but the architect, by chance an Old Cryptian, Rob Baggot, suggested that to do so would result in treating more of the staff than the animals. Nevertheless most of the four exterior walls were retained and it has seen much action since then.

A stone monument once stood at this crossroad in Brockworths, but as Ermin Street began to experience more than casual village traffic it was moved from the middle of the road. The heavy circular base lay for years at the foot of one of the forge walls and when we began our renovations the Parish Council asked if it could be moved to a safer and more public place. I agreed and at some point it was moved – and that was the last I saw of it. No doubt it is in a safe place, probably adorning an old councillor's garden somewhere! The little surgery grew rapidly and became a bustling place with many new clients joining the practice.

At the time of the Falklands conflict, Pam Profit, the wife of a high-ranking officer at neighbouring RAF Innsworth, was the practice secretary. When she joined the practice she knew that at some time in the future her husband would be moved to another station, but that was unlikely to be for a number of years. It was disappointing when she broke the unexpected news to us that their move to another part of the country, where her husband would be responsible for running his own base, was imminent. I know that Pam truly regretted leaving the practice after just eighteen months, but she was determined to find the best replacement with the minimum of bother to me. She advertised the post, contacted and interviewed the applicants, and made the final choice. She then brought her successful candidate to the surgery for an introduction and official approval.

Enter Joan Moat, a mature lady with excellent office skills and a polite and friendly manner. She was completely satisfactory for the position and was duly appointed. I suspect that Pam recognised that she possessed other qualities that made her perfect for the job. Joan always offered encouragement and advice, and was often a shoulder for a young nurse to cry on. As principal of the practice my involvement in this important arena of practice management was limited to sorting out the odd problem a male vet assistant might have, and this was usually done over a pint in the local. Joan was the mother of three grown-up children and married to Horace. I rarely, if ever, mentioned my efforts at jumping from a plane to him. Horace had been a true Para and a sergeant major in the regiment. He had parachuted into Normandy on D-Day and spent the remainder of the war battling his way across France. After almost two decades with us, I suspect that Mrs Moat wondered what her position and job description was in the practice. By the time Joan retired she was assumed, among other titles, to be the practice secretary, practice manager, personal assistant, legal and social adviser but, to most members of staff, she was Auntie Joan.

For most of this financially demanding decade by hook and by crook we stayed on even keel. The practice grew, expanded and thrived. The hours were long and tiring, but nearly always happy and rewarding and there was usually something to smile about. However, towards the end of the 1980s we went through a particularly sticky patch that I shall remember all my days. We could easily have gone bust. We were to some extent victims of our own success. I am sure that this is an over-used phrase in the business world but it was related, if not the cause, of our problems and we needed the support of the bank.

The small animal side of the practice was growingly rapidly and becoming ever more sophisticated. The need to invest in new equipment, employ more staff and provide bigger premises in which to house them had become paramount. The bank, as usual, was happy to finance the project and we could not foresee any problems. The architect drew up the plans, the builder extended the surgery, and we bought our new equipment, but we were close to the limit of our loan arrangements.

What we could not have predicted was that bank interest rates were about to go through the roof, and suddenly everyone wanted to be paid at once. After we had settled our account with the architect, the planners, the builders and the solicitors, it was time once more to pay the Inland Revenue and the VAT man. There were, of course, the electricity and gas bills, drug bills and a seemingly endless bundle of other demands to pay, but, most important of all, the staff had to be paid.

There were two factors aggravating our problems. The tightening of the economy meant that a large number of our own fees were not being paid. Our difficulties came to light when Joan discovered, to our embarrassment, that one of our cheques had bounced. Having reached the limit of our overdraft arrangement and marginally exceeded it, the bank decided to apply their new rules and their interest rates shot up from 18 per cent to 32.4 per cent.

I thought it was financial extortion verging on the criminal. Joan spent most of the next few weeks on the telephone negotiating with the latest business banking manager. Each week there seemed to be another unfamiliar face who claimed to be our new bank manager, but they all spoke the same impersonal language. It was thanks to Joan's coolness and negotiating skills that we kept afloat despite every new £1,000 loan costing us a £100 arrangement fee. If ever there was money for old rope! I had one option to escape from the bank's clutches, and reluctantly cashed in all my life insurance policies and then started them all over again.

I was sad in some respects to part with the bank that I had been with since my student days, but clearly loyalty now meant nothing. The days of Mr Mainwaring and the customer/local bank manager relationship were almost over, but I was pleased to move the practice account to the little branch of the Yorkshire Bank in Gloucester where we still felt that local customers had some relevance. In a very short time I had learnt that:

    Turn over is vanity
    Profit is reality
    Cash flow is sanity

I'll never need reminding of that. I needed no reminding either that I would soon be fifty.

CHAPTER EIGHT

M99: THE ANAESTHETIC FROM HELL

In the early 1960s, while I was beavering away at veterinary science in Liverpool, two research chemists concocted a drug which was labelled M99. It was chemically related to morphine but was 80,000 times more powerful. They called the substance etorphine hydrochloride. Combined with the powerful sedative acepromazine it was, and still is, marketed under the name of Immobilon. It is a very potent anaesthetic.

Its use today in the UK is restricted for use in dart guns for capturing and restraining large wild animals like deer and zoo animals. The procedures for emergency medical treatment should anyone be unfortunate enough to be scratched with a contaminated needle or receive a small eye splash are rigorously enforced today. The consequences of accidently injecting yourself are too scary to think about. The tiniest amount of the drug injected will very quickly cause dizziness, a drop in blood pressure, respiratory depression, cyanosis, loss of consciousness and death; quite an unpleasant way to go.

On a brighter note, by 1968 it was being advertised and promoted as the state-of-the-art convenience anaesthetic for use in horses and donkeys. A different and less potent version was available for use in dogs, but this was used on a much smaller scale. At the time it was launched by the pharmaceutical company, none of us vets realised just how serious self-injection of a small amount could be, and I do mean a small amount; the liquid film adhering to a used needle was enough to cause a life-threatening emergency. The attraction was that it was so convenient to use. A small volume of intravenous Immobilon was all that was required to put a horse of any size to the ground and allow quite extensive surgical procedures to be carried out. At the end of the operation, when you wanted the horse back on its feet, a similar volume of the antidote marketed under the name of Revivon was given by the same route and within minutes the horse would be standing, and amazingly often looking for food. It was not a perfect anaesthetic by any means and the much preferred technique of delivering anaesthetic gases directly to the patient via an endotracheal tube were vastly superior. The problem for most practices which were not essentially equine practices was that they did not carry out a sufficient number of general anaesthetics to justify the large financial expense of the more elaborate equipment. For the average practitioner involved in the welfare of a range of large animals, Immobilon seemed to be an injection too good to be true. It was certainly an improvement on some of the techniques still being used at the time.

One popular method was to force the horse to breathe chloroform vapour by putting a head-collar on the patient containing a sponge that fitted close to the nostrils. The liquid chloroform vaporised and the patient inhaled it. When sufficient had been taken in the horse fell over and remained anaesthetised, aided by an assistant who juggled with the sponge on or off the nostrils throughout the operation. At the end of the procedure the horse breathed clean air once more and gradually rose to its feet. Chloroform is an anaesthetic with a very small safety margin and not infrequently the patient did not get back on its feet. I recall seeing this procedure used on a regular routine basis as a young vet. Immobilon was at least an improvement on this. The patient was generally safe even though for the vet the procedure was fraught with danger. We simply were not aware of how dangerous the substance was until the first tragedy involving a veterinary surgeon occurred.

At the time of the incident, in the '70s, it was still customary to start the day on the farm wearing a clean brown freshly pressed smock-coat, the same style as the ones we had worn at Vet School. This particular young vet had gone along to a farm to carry out a routine castration of a colt. He drew up the calculated dose of Immobilon from his kit in the boot of his car and slipped the syringe and unprotected needle into the top pocket of his smock-coat. He approached the frisky young horse and as he did so the colt reared.

It was a situation that most vets involved with horses have experienced on one occasion or another. The natural response is to lift your arms to protect your face, which is what he did, and on bringing his arms down again his wrist was pierced by the needle and some Immobilon was injected. He was quickly incapacitated by the drug and tried desperately to reach his car in the hope of administering the antidote, Revivon. Had he succeeded his life may have been saved, but he died before he could reach the car.

The tragedy resulted in a huge amount of publicity in the veterinary press and started the alarm bells ringing. In hindsight it could have been argued that the vet had been careless in failing to apply the protective plastic cover to the needle of a loaded hypodermic syringe, and this omission led to the accidental injection. Quite right too, but I doubt if there is a single vet who works regularly with animals who has never accidentally pricked him or herself with a hypodermic needle. During the following weeks the veterinary press was full of alarming related reports of everyday experiences from vet practitioners. Several described the effect of an accidental needle puncture as they scrambled over a stile. The rapid onset of dizziness was a frequent reminder that the plastic cap of the needle was in the other pocket.

The one positive thing that resulted from this sad fatality was that it was instantly clear how dangerous it was to use this anaesthetic at all. The moral conclusion was that if you continued to use it, now being aware of the dangers, on your own head be it. The problem was that it was so useful, particularly in emergency situations, that most vets did continue to use it. The safety precautions leading up to the actual injection of the drug and the care given to the disposal of any needle that had come near it was like nothing we had ever experienced before. But regardless of all these precautions the result of accidental injection was still a possibility, and strict ground rules were laid down. The recommended antidote to etorphine in people is a drug called naloxone and it is marketed in phials as Narcan.

It was customary (and today essential) to take an assistant, preferably a trusted, experienced veterinary nurse, with you to any operation where Immobilon was to be used. At the commencement of the proceedings she was reminded once more of the emergency procedures if, heaven forbid, it became necessary. If instructed, it was essential for the nurse to inject without hesitation at least one phial containing 2ml of Narcan deeply into a muscle. The vet's backside was the site of choice, and although vets generally do have a wonderful sense of humour, you can appreciate that for various reasons practical rehearsals were out of the question. I often wondered, as I approached a horse's jugular vein with the Immobilon in hand, whether if things suddenly went pear-shaped the nurse would actually muster the courage to pull the boss' jeans down and ram the naloxone needle into my posterior. No doubt the odd nurse would have relished the opportunity! I continued to use the drug throughout the 1970s and '80s, usually for well-planned routine procedures in the horse, such as castrations and dental operations, and of course I did use it during unexpected emergencies. It is strange how so many of these occur at night. When the telephone rang late one evening I was surprised to hear Richard Pullen, a local dairy farmer whose wife, Judy, was the current Master of the Cotswold Hunt, on the other end of the line asking me *not* to attend a cow going down with mile fever but something far more dramatic. Richard spoke in a despondent tone.

'There's been a bit of a disaster, Ivor. Judy's mare has been hit by a car or something and I don't think there is much you can do. Come and have a look and see what you think – but I expect you'll be putting her down.'

I reached the farm a few minutes later. The beautiful black mare, Moffet, was still standing and they had managed to walk her the short distance from the Badgeworth road, where she had been hit, to a small paddock nearer Reddings Farm. She stood motionless in the darkness, a dark mare lit from behind by a very bright moon. I approached her quietly and spoke her name, then moved to the front of her and gulped as I looked at the gaping wound to her chest for the first time. I stepped back, aghast at the enormity of the cavity that I was looking into. It was astonishing that she was still on her feet, but it made my examination of her that much easier. Richard stood next to me. His manner was uncustomarily sharp and abrupt.

'I don't want any messin' about, Ivor, if you think you can save her have a go, otherwise put her down now.' Quite a challenge from one of your best clients, but at least I knew where I stood. I decided to have a go. The wound was huge but I could find no evidence that the thoracic cavity itself had been entered. Through my stethoscope I could hear every abnormal respiratory sound that had ever been described in one of my university text books ringing in my ear. She had suffered immense pulmonary contusion, and the tearing of lung tissue was probably present everywhere in her deep chest. In view of what had happened, this was both inevitable and expected. It might take a long time, but, eventually, I thought she could recover from the damage that she had sustained.

Having made the decision to operate, I returned to my surgery and collected an enormous pack of sterile instruments, metres of catgut and synthetic nylon suture material, boxes of cotton wool and sterile swabs, bottles of antibiotic, steroids and local anaesthetic, and hoped that I had not forgotten an essential item. I apprehensively removed the polystyrene boxes of Immobilon, Revivon and Narcan from the locked poison cabinet. How I wished at that moment for the anaesthetic equipment my Liverpool lecturers had used at Leahurst not so many years before. Their technique was so smooth and rehearsed: sedation of the patient, anaesthetic induction with thiopentone, tracheal intubation, administration of a halothane/oxygen mixture and controlled anaesthesia until the job was done. The thought of a student observing those operations with a syringe of Narcan in hand, awaiting the opportunity to jab it into the rear end of a lecturer, was rather comical, but this was no time for joking. I loaded everything into the back of my faithful little MG and set off.

Back at the farm, at least the 'operating theatre' resembled more than I had been taught to expect under field conditions by the Leahurst teaching staff. A deep layer of clean straw bedding was surrounded by straw bales. One was to be used as my operating table while the others had been arranged in tiers at varying distances, apparently to provide seating accommodation for the small crowd of observers that had arrived during my absence. Nor could I complain about a lack of light – the spotlights on all the farm vehicles were being put to good use. Richard and Judy led their mare to the centre of the operating area.

It had become a little theatrical and I was aware of the hushed audience as I felt for the pulsating jugular vein in her neck. She hardly reacted as I pierced the vessel and injected the Immobilon, giving the largest dose I felt she could take in her shocked state. Just moments later she staggered and crumpled to the floor, and as she collapsed fresh blood and serum spurted from the injuries as the uppermost weight of her body put immense pressure on the wounds. I must have spent the next ten minutes and probably longer cleaning and debriding the traumatised area. Bits of metal, glass and gravel seemed to be everywhere embedded in the skin.

The repair eventually began. For the next hour I lay on the straw almost head to head with my patient, removing strips of tattered and torn muscles and dissecting back to tissues I hoped would remain viable despite the trauma of the impact. I had become oblivious to the onlookers until a hushed gasp reminded me they were still watching. I had released a large piece of bone that had been part of her sternum and was better dissected free than left to cause a problem later. I teased it out and remarked to Richard, 'I'm sure she can manage without this bit', and placed it on the operating table. Putting the jigsaw back together took a long time. Scores of catgut sutures later resulted in the semblance of an intact-looking brisket. To reach the lower sternal area we manoeuvered her gently on to her back and supported her with more bales. I was glad that so many strong chaps were instantly available. The operation continued into the second hour and was free of unexpected complications.

She was at last back in one piece and I was able to look down on a line of nylon skin sutures that appeared to go on forever. If it was not a work of art I thought it looked pretty good anyway. I was glad to be back on my feet, but I was much more anxious to see my patient back on hers. The decks were cleared of buckets of soiled surgical dressings, drapes, instruments and the surgical bales. The final treatments for the evening were the antibiotics, the steroids, the analgesics and anti-tetanus injections. Satisfied I could do no more I felt again for the jugular, injected the Revivon and waited. The next few minutes seemed an eternity. Then she lifted her head and slowly rose to her feet. Although looking slightly perplexed, she was soon acknowledging the presence of her owners.

I had a last look at her over the stable door before enjoying a well-deserved nightcap with Richard. He now resembled his more relaxed self and the conversation had moved on from horses to Gloucester Rugby. That particular night was a memorable one for many reasons. It was an example of what could be achieved under field conditions with the minimum of equipment and the appropriate training. It took about two months for Moffet to recover completely from the dreadful accident and I saw a great deal of her during this time. Two years later she produced a fine colt foal, Soup Dragon, who represented Britain overseas on four occasions. This was a story with a joyful ending.

Sadly, there were occasions when things did not end so well. Donkeys have been part of farming and commercial life in the Cotswolds for centuries, but in more recent times they have become increasingly popular as companion animals. Approaching maturity, the donkey stallion normally requires castration, and using Immobilon as the anaesthetic of convenience was common throughout the 1960s and '70s. The donkey responded in a similar manner to the horse with regard to its anaesthetic effect and the immediate response to the Revivon injections was similar, initially. Sometimes, for complex biochemical reasons that I won't try to explain here because I have never fully understood them myself, the complete anaesthetic recovery suddenly stops and the donkey returns to an unstable wobbly state. This could safely be reversed once more with further treatment with Revivon, and the owner was instructed to check frequently on the donkey in the hours following the operation.

'Phone if you are concerned in any way', we said.

You could bet on that call coming at midnight followed by another trip to a stable on the side of a Cotswold hill in the pouring rain. It was not always like that of course, but those are the nights that you remember.

The Smith family at Pirton Court, who are not relatives as far as I am aware, had farmed in Churchdown for several generations. They were dairy farmers in the '70s and Howard Smith, one of the partners in the family business, was at about this time Master of the Cotswold Hunt. When I first visited the farm and met the family it was difficult to avoid Granddad Smith. He was well into his nineties and, whenever I met him on the farm, the guessing game began.

'How old do you think I am?' He would ask.

'Seventy-four?' I offered on the first occasion, in case he was actually eighty-three. In fairness the old man did not look any older.

'No, older than that', was the usual reply.

'Okay then, eighty-three?'

'Getting nearer', he teased.

And so the game went on until we finally reached his true age. His grandson, Mervin, shared the same family interest in horses. As an amateur jockey he had suffered severe chest injuries from a racing fall in the 1960s, but had bounced back and married Val, one of Gloucester's prestigious Miss Gloucesters. Mervin owned a young colt that he asked me to cut, 'cutting' being a common usage in horse circles for castration. 'Gelding the horse' is the expression used in polite company. At the start of this particular operation, the lively colt was referred to by one of the farm's labourers as one that "bout time 'e 'ad is nackers off", another frequently used expression in farming circles.

I was happy to carry out the operation no matter how it was described, and armed with the now customary polystyrene boxes of Immobilon, Revivon, Narcan and accompanied by a trusted nurse, I arrived at the farm one crisp April morning. I carried the drugs, the nurse carried the instruments and other equipment and someone else carried the essential bucket of hot water, soap and towel. Mervin led the colt out to the edge of one of the large flat fields at Pirton Court.

I ran through the emergency routine with my nurse and hoped she would not be chatting should I require her immediate attention whilst using the Immobilon. We were further assisted by one of the farmworkers, a local chap who was normally responsible for milking the cows, but, like most fellows at that time who had grown up on a farm, could competently handle most animals. He stood on one side of the colt's head with Mervin on the other. I raised the jugular vein and inserted a large needle. Venous blood flowed from it and I attached the syringe containing the Immobilon, and injected. With that nerve-racking part over, the operation could begin, everyone a little less tense now that the dreaded syringe and needle was safely shut away. The patient stumbled to the ground in the expected manner and over the next few minutes became increasingly relaxed as the drug took effect.

The straw bale operating table was draped, the instruments arranged neatly on it, and with the uppermost leg roped, pulled forward and restrained by our helpers, the nurse had the honour of washing, cleaning and sterilising the patient's scrotum and surrounding area while I scrubbed up. That done to her satisfaction, she peeled a blade from its sterile packet and I clipped it into the scalpel handle. I kneeled beside the hind legs, grasped the lower testicle and incised over it. It took seconds to isolate the organ and to reveal the vascular spermatic cord. My nurse passed me the instrument that had been designed a century before: the emasculator. This particular model, made in brilliantly shiny stainless steel, was very much younger, but probably not a great deal more efficient, than the original version. It was designed to cut through and crush the spermatic cord in one operation, and to ensure this was done efficiently the tool was held in situ for a good three minutes before being removed. That's a long time when you are holding a long, heavy instrument very still and your arms begin to complain. The cunning vet directs the jaws of the instrument to the correct anatomical position and passes the other draped end to the nurse to hold and tells her to release it when the time is up. The routine was then repeated on the uppermost testicle.

There is a right way and a wrong way of applying the instrument, and if used the wrong way round there will be problems. The business end of the emasculator that cuts and crushes does so in one direction only. Thus, if the crushing takes place below the cutting the result is a severe haemorrhage that can be difficult to control. There are two small wingnuts that are used to dismantle the metal components after use for cleaning and sterilising. To ensure that we never got it wrong, our lecturers in surgery gave us the following memorable advice: 'Always make sure the nuts are facing the nuts.'

Having checked to ensure there was no unexpected haemorrhage, the surgical site was dusted with an antibiotic powder and the area cleaned of blood. Once the routine anti-tetanus and antibiotic injections had been given, and the restraints on the leg removed, it was time to get the patient back on his feet. I injected the appropriate volume of Revivon and waited for him to scramble to his feet, look around slightly bewildered and then begin to graze quietly. After several minutes nothing happened. There was a slight increase in his respiratory rate and once more I listened to his heart through my stethoscope. I could find no reason for the lack of response. To remove any impression that I was getting concerned I joked, 'I think he must be too comfortable down there.' Mervin had attached a long rope lead to his head-collar and was crouching over him. Perhaps our patient became aware of the presence of other horses neighing in nearby fields, and he decided to get up. Not slowly, but like a bat out of hell. Fortunately, Mervin was hanging on to the head-collar, which was just as well, otherwise within minutes that thoroughbred colt would have been in Gloucester. How he hung on I'll never know – it was a brave effort and at times resembled a bucking bronco; we expected him to leap on to his back and off again, ride bareback, sidesaddle and facing backwards. The entertainment finally ended halfway through the second lap of the huge field as they decelerated to a halt. I was so relieved when it finally stopped and both my client and my patient were still in one piece. They both made a speedy recovery.

We returned to the surgery and, over a cup of strong coffee, were able to see the funny side of an event that could easily have ended in disaster. I swore to my nurse that I would never use that damned anaesthetic on a thoroughbred horse ever again. But I did. It happened not too long after the last escapade.

Mrs Delia Beltram was a very well-known lady in the local horse world, and probably farther afield too. She had numerous horses that were kept in various parts of the county and at any time a disaster requiring veterinary attention was always on the cards, but even with Mrs Beltram's track record it seemed extremely unlikely that a routine castration of one of them would cause any problems.

This particular young stallion was kept at stables in Sandhurst Lane on the outskirts of Gloucester and, with the boot of my car packed with the all the usual essentials, my nurse and I made our way there early one pleasant spring afternoon. It was around the time of the annual Gold Cup Meeting at Cheltenham, and as we travelled along the northern city bypass scores of race-goers were travelling in the opposite direction. I wished I could have been one of them.

We had been at the stables looking for Mrs Beltram for about twenty minutes when we started to wonder if she had forgotten the arrangement. Then she appeared around the corner of a building pushing a wheelbarrow heaped with horse manure. The next half-hour was spent searching for a suitable site to carry out the operation, borrowing bales of straw from other stable owners, finding a suitable bucket for the essential hot water, soap and towel, and a head-collar that fitted the horse to my satisfaction. Eventually, I stood next to the stallion's head and steeled myself for administering the Immobilon injection. In my mind I knew that if ever there was going to be a jeans down day, this was going to be it.

Surprisingly, the anaesthesia and the operation went more smoothly than I had dared hope and in no time at all I was preparing to bring the stallion round and get him back on his feet. We removed every conceivable obstacle from the small paddock that I had used as the operating arena. I injected the Revivon. I had no idea about this horse's pedigree, but I would bet his ancestors had won the Derby and the Grand National. He rose to his feet in a flash but unfortunately Mrs Beltram was no Mervin, and after two laps of the paddock he cleared the low fence, charged at the boundary hedge, jumped and cleared it with ease and disappeared up Sandhurst Lane. I had never lost a patient in this manner before. I suspected that the owner expected me to go and find him.

He had a head start but we knew in which direction he was going. My nurse dived into the car next to me and we tore off, closely followed by Mrs Beltram in her banger. Not for the first time in my professional career I felt I had recreated a scene from the *Keystone Kops*. We soon reached the top of the lane and the busy junction with St Oswald's Road and its dual carriageway. There was no sign of the stallion, but fortunately there were numerous pedestrians around. Anxiously I asked one of them:

'Have you seen a horse in the last few minutes?' The first responder looked at us as though we were daft and replied, 'No'. The second asked what the rider looked like and what colour the horse was. I was about to say that it was a riderless horse and the prominent colour by now would be a dark red patch somewhere in the region of the hind legs, when a third person approached.

'Are you looking for a horse?' the lady asked.

'Yes!'

'Oh, I'm so glad. I saw one a short while ago running towards the Tewkesbury road.'

There was hardly time to thank her as we sped off again. At least now we knew that our patient was probably somewhere between Gloucester and Tewkesbury, but at the rate he was travelling he could have been halfway to Worcester by now.

In the distance we could hear the sound of an emergency services' siren. I glanced at my nurse and, half-whispering through a dry mouth, queried, 'Do you reckon that could be anything to do with us?' She didn't reply but I suspected we were both envisaging a line of dented cars trying to dodge a runaway horse. A few miles down the road we neared a smallholding with stables that I knew well. Nearby were the blue flashing lights of a police car that had arrived shortly before us. I braked sharply and swerved into the yard. As I got out of the car I was greeted by a policeman, who asked, 'Does this horse belong to you, sir?' Perhaps he had noticed that I was still covered in congealed blood and deduced that I may in some way be related to the horse.

'Well, he's not exactly mine, officer', I replied, unconvincingly.

I was praying that Mrs Beltram's old jalopy had not broken down, as it often did, and that she would soon arrive to claim her horse. I was about to explain to the officer that I had been operating on the horse when he decided to run away, when Mrs Beltram pulled into the yard and twice loudly sounded her horn. My prayers were answered and I was spared having to offer my explanation to the police. Delia, as usual, did all the talking, but did not tell him who I was. The officer eventually turned to me and commented:

'It looks as though the horse is injured, sir, I think we should call a vet.'

I considered explaining to him that, well, actually I *was* a vet and I *was* operating on the patient when suddenly he — but it all sounded so unbelievable that it was far simpler to say, 'Thank you, officer, I'll take over and do all that is necessary.' He turned off the blue flashing lights and drove off, probably wondering if he was suffering from overwork.

The next day I carried out a post-operative check on my patient, something that was not normally necessary but on this occasion, as it was about six miles from where the operation had started, I felt that there were mitigating circumstances. He showed no adverse signs following his immediate post-operative physiotherapy, but for my own wellbeing as much as his, I would not recommend it.

I am sure the reader will be glad to know that Immobillon is not commonly used today. Restraining wild animals via a dart gun is its main use. It does not take much stretch of the imagination to appreciate that there are other uses for a drug mix that can be used for other purposes. Its use as a means of quickly terminating life is an obvious one. Not surprisingly, Immobilon is at times used today for carrying out euthanasia. Once again it has to be described as something that can be used when nothing better is available.

Most of us watch the news on television and I'm sure some can remember the interest in recent times of the whale, a huge Northern Bottlenose, which became stranded in the River Thames in London. At some point it became obvious to the vets monitoring the situation that the whale was dying and when he began to convulse it was decided on humane grounds that it was time for euthanasia. How do you put to sleep an animal of such huge proportions? It is frighteningly easy with just a small bottle of Immobilon. The appropriate dose is calculated by estimating the length of the animal and injecting 4ml of the substance for each 1½ metres through a 25cm needle. Sadly, there was no need to administer it, and the Prince of Whales, as one newspaper christened him, died after one final episode of convulsing.

With such a potent weapon available, it was only a matter of time before misuse of the drug would be involved in a story that could have come straight from the pen of Agatha Christie. If you desire to murder your wife, and you are a vet who has easy access to the poison, what a wonderful storyline this would make. If the vet is deeply in debt and stands to collect £180,000 of his wife's life insurance money, then the story gets more intriguing. This actually happened in 1994, when the wife of a Staffordshire vet was found dead in suspicious circumstances. Traces of Immobilon were found in her body and her husband soon became the chief suspect. Although unexplained needle puncture marks were found on her feet, her husband was accused of murdering her by spiking her orange juice with Immobilon. With evidence like this stacked against you, you cannot possibly be innocent. That is what the jury believed when they found him guilty, and clearly the judge did not like the vet too much, referring to him as 'the most evil, selfish and criminally callous man' he had ever sentenced. Unsurprisingly, the vet was handed down a life sentence in 1995.

Well, he was guilty, wasn't he? No, actually he was not. Everyone seemed to believe so until a hand-written note, signed by the deceased, was found between the pages of a copy of the faithful old *Veterinary Record*. It read, 'I leave you absolutely nothing but this note – if you find it in time.' In 1998 the Court of Appeal quashed the conviction and the vet was freed. The case was summed up by a QC who aptly described it thus, 'The prosecution say this was murder made to look like suicide. We say it was most likely suicide made to look like murder.' Tragically, this sad case would not be an isolated suicide brought about by the administration of a tiny dose of Immobilon. The deaths of numerous vets would be recorded over the following years.

CHAPTER NINE

NEVER WORK WITH CHILDREN OR ANIMALS

Media performers, whether they are related to television, radio, the cinema or theatre, strongly advise that it is best to steer clear of animals and children. Both are guaranteed to embarrass you and to expose your weaknesses. This is excellent advice, but naturally in my case it was only possible to try and stay clear of the youngsters for a little while. Nevertheless, talking to large groups of children in classrooms and halls at Cub and Brownie meetings was always enjoyable. I soon learned to treat the children as mini-adults and I expected that respect to be reciprocated. They definitely seemed to resent being told childish jokes. This one did not go down well:

Have you heard the story about the dog that had to go to the vet's hospital because he became ill after eating some daffodil bulbs? The worried owner asked the vet if his dog would get better. 'Yes', said the vet, 'but he's very poorly and will have to stay in my hospital for a long time.' 'Oh dear', said the owner, 'When can he come home?' The vet thought for a moment before replying, 'Oh, he should be out in the spring!'

It is a wonderful feeling when your audience is amused by the punchline and have difficulty staying on their seats, and nothing more deflating when the joke falls flat. There is nothing worse than looking at a sea of expressionless children's faces, and wondering what they are thinking. Children are gifted with a natural desire for learning, and at times I have been inwardly embarrassed by the simplest of questions relating to such things as the animals' senses and the behaviour of our pets that seem too mundane for the professional, myself included, to give a second thought to.

'Why do dogs bury bones?'

'Why doesn't our dog bury bones?'

'Can cats and dogs see colours?'

'What about the horse, cow, guinea pig, mouse, snake? What colours can they see?'

'You came to our house and put our cat to sleep. Did he go to heaven?'

At the time I probably thought, 'Ask me about the need for vitamin A and its biological role in the animal body and I'll blind you with science.' One thing I learned was to listen to the children. They are too young to be anyone's fool.

By the time I retired, the youngsters I had met in the 1960s had become the mums and dads bringing their own children to the surgery, and in some cases their grandchildren too. It is astonishing to believe that the little girl whose mice disappeared under the Crudwell surgery floorboards in 1966 is now in her forties. Time really does go by very quickly. With luck she will have forgotten that whole tragic occasion. I remember it well.

Vet School training in the 1960s concentrated on the surgery, medicine and husbandry of, in descending size, the horse, cow, sheep, pig, dog, cat and poultry. That was ample for me. Rabbits were given some consideration, but it was expected that the ones we were being taught to care for would eventually end up on a plate. How things have changed. The practising veterinary surgeon today is also expected to deal competently with the cuddly bunnies, guinea pigs, chinchillas, hamsters, rats, gerbils, mice, cold-water fish, tropical fish, tortoises, terrapins, budgerigars, canaries, parrots, the Vietnamese pot-bellied pig and the back yard fowl. Today, any creature we dare to share our homes with is referred to as a companion animal. When I qualified, these latter animals were considered exotic pets. 'Bugsy', the house rabbit, is an exotic pet? Not any more. These days he's part of the family and his medicine and surgery is expected to be high on the vet's list of priority matters. Not surprisingly there has been both a need and a trend towards veterinary practitioner specialisation. Having said that, I don't think the previous generations of vets fared too badly using our knowledge of basic medicine and a modicum of common sense, even if at times it did land us in some sticky situations.

I have yet to mention our third group of exotic pets; the wildlife patients. One Saturday afternoon, I was watching a Wales *v.* England rugby contest on television. Nearing the end of a nail-biting second half the telephone rang. The desperate lady on the end of the line, whose husband I bet was watching the rugby, was adamant that a frightened blackbird she had rescued was in need of immediate veterinary attention. I left the game with Wales creeping ahead thanks to a disputed penalty goal and headed for the surgery. To appear professional – even on a Saturday afternoon in the middle of a rugby game – I donned a clean white coat.

The lady thanked me for seeing the bird so swiftly and deposited the bird-containing wicker basket on to the examination table. I carefully opened the top and the frantic patient made the most of its opportunity to escape. What the lady had failed to tell me was that her husband had retrieved the bird from a pool of sump oil in their garage. This became pretty obvious when the bird hit the recently decorated Persil-white ceiling, struck a wall, splattered against another wall, and then another. By the time I caught him, my consulting room looked like a scene from the *Black and White Minstrel Show* and I looked like one of the singers.

While my Saturday afternoon nurse cleansed the bird in detergent and prepared it for release the next day, I queried, not for the first time, if the public ever asked themselves how this free service was financed. My nurse told me to stop being stingey, cheer up and go home and watch the rest of the rugby. An hour or so later I went home and Angela gave me more bad news: the final score of the international game. I didn't think about the event again until I signed a cheque a week or so later for the decorator, 'for removing oil before applying three coats of brilliant white emulsion'.

In the Gloucester area, it was difficult to escape for long the presence of the city's famous rugby club. Gloucester has produced more than its fair share of superstars, but for some mysterious and inexplicable reason it is the usual practice for the England management to overlook them for selection for international duties. Mike Burton, however, was a player the selectors could not ignore. He was a frequent visitor to the surgery in the '70s with his young family and their pets. One evening he came in with a lame guinea pig. The upper part of one hind leg was very swollen and painful. Through the swelling the broken ends of a fractured femur were easily palpated. Mike, at this time in the pre-professional rugby era, had still to earn his fortune and was pleased to opt for the most economical treatment I suggested. Actually what I advised was perfectly suitable, and where a limb can be immobilised for a couple of weeks, the bones of a healthy guinea pig will heal rapidly. A state-of-the-art material that was claimed to be a spin-off from the space research industry was a plastic gauze material that had the strange property of being malleable in very hot water but when cooled to room temperature it stiffened and seemed to have the strength of steel. It was a welcome opportunity to use it for the first time, and it worked well. Removing it, however, was a problem as each mesh had to be snipped through individually before the cast could be removed, but at least it prevented the patient gnawing through it and removing it prematurely.

Mike enjoyed his animals and probably still does. I wouldn't refer to him as a frustrated farmer but he took pride in a large group of calves that he cared for on a small farm at Shurdington, a few miles outside Cheltenham. I often went there to treat the usual problems of young cattle: scouring, respiratory disease and the odd lameness. I suppose you could liken many of their ailments to those of young local rugby players on a Sunday morning. But Mike was no longer a local player.

One cold, wet winter evening I turned off the main road and approached his farm buildings along a newly laid concrete drive. It was the sort of surface Lewis Hamilton might have had problems with, and within minutes I failed to negotiate a slippery bend that had been treated with copious amounts of storm water and cattle slurry, and the rear wheels of the little MG slid off the track. I emerged reluctantly from the cockpit and in no time at all was welcomed by farmer Burton appearing from the gloom by torchlight. I was greeted with, 'Evening Ivor! Sorry about this, don't get out.' I was expecting a helpful tractor with a tow rope to appear, but I was very soon aware of things happening at the rear of the car, and a lot of grunting. The back end lifted and the MG moved sideways a little, enough for the wheels to be back on solid concrete. 'Lord', I prayed, as one does in an extreme emergency. 'Please don't let him be ruptured, well not on this occasion.'

Mike was destined to collect his first England cap within hours. Alone, he had lifted the car from the mire: an astonishing feat of strength. Bravo, but what if he had acquired a scrotal hernia? I could imagine the headlines in the *Cheltenham Echo*, 'Vet and Rugby star both in the slurry', or words to that effect. He survived unblemished and turned out at Twickenham the following Saturday afternoon and I avoided being one of the most unpopular Gloucester rugby supporters ever. I cannot imagine how the Shed would have responded. They probably would have conjured up something like, 'Thanks to vet, Burton needs more support.'

Mike has a wicked sense of humour and one of the funniest books I have ever read is his imaginary autobiography, *Have Balls Will Travel*. It was a relief to know that they did not travel far that awful night. Mike was a powerful chap, but he was not the largest rugby star to squeeze into my surgery. That honour must go to our Welsh international forward Ben Edwards, who also lived in Shurdington for many years. When he brought his Dachshund dog to surgery, the little fellow trotted in while his owner barely managed to manoeuvre his vast frame through the doorway after him. He was one of rugby's many gentle giants.

It would be easy to digress into tales concerning other Gloucestershire sporting characters and their antics with their animals, but I shan't do so here. In the days before professionalism, so many talented local sportspersons were denied the opportunity of a career in sport, assuming of course that that was what they wanted. Old Richian Michael (Mick) Sparey was one of them. His Saturday winters were spent tenaciously on local muddy rugby fields, but his summer cricketing skills were generally well acknowledged as being exceptional.

Mick's wife, Jacqui, was a Denmark Grammar School old girl and a teacher at Gloucester's Tredworth Road junior school. Her teaching enthusiasm extended to after-school activities and the school's Natural History Society was one of her interests. I was pleased to accept her invitation to give an animal-orientated talk to the youngsters. They had been asked to bring along their pets to the meeting where 'Mr Smith will spend an hour or so giving advice to the young members on their care and management.'

At 4.10 p.m. one dark winter's afternoon, I arrived at the school and met my audience and their furry friends. Actually, one of them wasn't that furry. In fact he looked quite smooth, exceptionally smooth. It was a snake, and in the confines of his 5lb jam jar, there seemed an awful lot of him. For some reason it crossed my mind that it could be a particularly lethal species, but he was safe enough while he remained in his jar. My lecture started and the hour that followed was immensely enjoyable.

I had demonstrated my small-animal handling skills and had given the appropriate advice on feeding and breeding them, and managed to avoid the usual unimaginable questions that only children could ask. Jacqui rose and thanked me for my attendance, but before I departed she begged me to answer the question that all the children were dying to ask: 'How does a vet handle a snake?' She failed to add, 'a snake of unknown origin and venom.'

I wished that the owner had by now left to attend his martial arts class. But he hadn't. As my blood pressure began to rise I could see the onlookers leaning forward in anticipation, and there seemed no alternative but to grapple with the creature. I picked up the jar and began to release the lid. The inhabitant knew something was happening and a spotted head peered over the rim. He had probably just received the first scent of human perspiration. I hoped he would not get too excited but within seconds he was everywhere. As he rose up there seemed to be yards of him still in the jar, and suddenly it occurred to me that if he got on to the floor there could be pandemonium as he wriggled across the classroom, and at that moment there was a fair chance of that happening. I definitely didn't want that to happen, so I grasped him just below his head as he emerged, which seemed to help him out of his jar, and suddenly I was holding a huge writhing snake. I yelled to the excited children that this was how you handled a lively snake, at the same time forcing his tail end back into the jar and vigorously encouraging the rest of the reluctant squirming body to follow. I finally slammed the lid on and screwed it tightly shut. I tried to smile and look composed. The amused owner grinned and explained to everyone that his metres of reptile was a harmless garter snake. Well, it did not look harmless to me.

I totally understand why we share our homes with dogs and cats, cuddly rabbits and guinea pigs, and occasionally a pony or donkey in the garden. I know that it takes all sorts and our world is a more interesting place as a result, but I have never really understood why anyone should choose to keep a snake or allow rats to wander around their lounge. But beauty lies in the eye of the beholder and I cannot deny the popularity of the pet rat.

One evening I heard screams coming from the waiting room. It was our receptionist and it sounded as though she were being attacked. We dashed to her aid and found her propped against a wall, her face the same colour as her white smock. A nurse passed her a glass of water and explained what had happened to us. It was the evening receptionist's first week and she had not yet grown accustomed to some of the unusual visitors to a vet's waiting room. After taking a particular client's particulars she asked for details of the pet brought in in a shoe box. She helpfully lifted the lid and was greeted by the inquisitive head of the biggest black rat she had ever seen in her life.

A shoe box, shopping bag, wicker fishing basket or wooden toolbox were often the customary ways of transporting pets to the surgery before the development of the strong plastic box in the '70s. The new type of plastic carrier was secure and hygienic and most could be easily cleaned and disinfected. One disadvantage to the vet could be the length of time it took to actually get the animal out of the box to examine it. I am certain that some surgery times were extended by at least half an hour as a result of owners struggling to open the box and persuade their pets to come out. Usually this was because a parent had brought the pet to surgery on an occasion when they were not accompanied by their smart child, who could release the lid in seconds. To be fair, some of the contraptions were designed so that unless you had a degree in Lego you would never succeed in releasing the animal. After one embarrassing occasion I was always reluctant to be too helpful in opening the carrier. Regrettably, they were not all made of high quality rigid unbreakable plastic, as I discovered one Sunday morning.

A sweet young girl had brought her bunny to surgery on her own, and with great determination lifted the plastic box and rabbit on to the examination table. She began to undo the first of the four clips that secured the lid but her fingers lacked the required strength. 'Shall I help?'

I volunteered, as I gripped the clip nearest me. It was certainly tough to open, and when it unclipped, it snapped off and was left in my hand. The young owner looked a little puzzled but I thought she would burst into tears when the second clip snapped off too. I really did not know what to say, so I shouted the first thing I could think of: 'Nurse!' My nurse raided the animal room, where she found and donated another plastic carrier to the youngster. It was an easy-for-the-vet-to-open-without-breaking-it type carrier. I said as little as possible and the young client went home happy with her pal in a smart new carrier.

The strong plastic box became the conventional and generally satisfactory way of transporting smaller animals, but there remains to this day, I am sure, the unconventional rat owner. Some of these love to enter the consulting room apparently without the patient and then at the last moment surprise the vet by producing him from under his jumper. Occasionally it was from under her jumper and I had to look away in case there was any prolonged difficulty extricating the inquisitive pet from the depths. On these unusual occasions you can bet at the end of the consultation the rat will be tucked back under the jumper or allowed to run up the owner's sleeve once more. Bizarrely, the deep relationship between owner and pet rat is usually genuine and at times quite touching, and despite what you might expect they rarely bite. A stranger handling them when they are unwell is sometimes the exception to this rule.

From time to time I have found myself somewhat reluctantly involved in the treatment of the pet fox. Many would argue that it is unnatural and cruel to try to domesticate the fox, but it is hard to explain that to a client who has had an apparently abandoned cub living with her for several weeks. In captivity the young animal has not learned to hunt and has become dependent on the owner for regular meals. When the owner is adamant that euthanasia of the young fox will not be considered as an option it leads to a tricky dilemma.

I found myself in this situation in the '80s when a young fox was brought to surgery wearing a collar and attached to a dog's lead. I knew the owner well as she was the fond owner of a German Shepherd dog. The fox cub had come into her possession as she drove to Churchdown one night. He had apparently been abandoned by his parents at the side of the road and was weak and sufficiently distressed to allow her to pick him up. At home, after a few days' rest and plenty of good food, he made a speedy recovery. But that was weeks ago and now it was too late to release him back into the wild with any realistic chance of survival. No doubt farmers would argue that he should have been destroyed in any case. The owner argued vehemently the other way and he remained her pet. Over the next year he grew accustomed to a daily domestic routine, which included walks around Churchdown on his lead. Most of the time he seemed to get on well with the German Shepherd he shared a home with, until, as he matured, he began to show some aggressive instincts towards the dog.

The distraught owner asked for my advice about the problem. I knew that discussing euthanasia would be pointless and I recommended that he was castrated before a more serious behavioural problem developed. While he was under the anaesthetic she was pleased to hear me suggest that I remove his scent glands at the same time. Only the owner knew how much the latter problem was, but if there is one smell I hate more than any other it is the smell of the fox. Why our dogs enjoy coming back home from a walk across fields smelling like a fox I shall never know. The scent glands in the true sense are not really glands at all. They are a pair of small sacs lying near the anal sphincter muscles in carnivores, and their walls are lined with a mixture of sebaceous and apocrine glands. The combination of this mixture of secretions produces an obnoxious smell. When the dog or the fox passes faeces, a small quantity is expelled and the process results in a form of territorial marking. It is not unusual of course for an excitable dog when he is being handled to squirt much larger quantities of this foul liquid over the vet.

The fox was admitted for surgery and I was about to enter a new learning curve on handling animals. His owner had gently popped him into a small kennel, but as soon as she left he reverted to his wild and natural preservation instincts. I had stroked his head on previous occasions when cradled in his owner's arms and as I talked quietly to him I attempted to give the same reassurance and hoped that he would remain still long enough for me to slip in a small painless subcutaneous injection of acetyl promazine. Once he was sufficiently sedated the rest of the procedures I intended to carry out would be quite routine.

I hardly saw him move as he whipped round and his slashing canine teeth opened an incision on my arm nearly 5cm long. This fellow had the strength of a dog and the agility of a cat. My nurse dressed my wrist and, once bitten, we took appropriate steps to avoid it happening again. Soon Mr Fox was sedated, relaxed and ready for the operating table. He went home with lines of sutures under his tail and between his legs.

When he arrived at the surgery ten days later to have the sutures removed he was easily given a sedative injection while cradled in his owner's arms and caused no problems that day. I was satisfied with his progress. We were both healing well.

The frequent opportunities that presented themselves to talk to children's groups meant that there were ample opportunities to discourage them from even considering having a wild animal as a pet. It is great fun to give them names and call a visiting pheasant to the garden Fudge, or the local squirrel that pinches the nuts from the bird feeder Charlie, but they do not make good pets. Grey squirrels sometimes created unexpected problems when they were brought to surgery with often relatively minor injuries that they had sustained in road accidents. Invariably it was mum accompanied by the children on their way home from school who found the injured animal. No doubt mum reassured the children that the nice vet would make the animal better. The vet in these cases could take just one course of action, and Charlie would be painlessly put to sleep. It is of course illegal to treat and to return grey squirrels to the wild. Explaining this to the kind family who came visiting the following day to see how Charlie was progressing was very hard.

There was never a problem explaining to other folk who brought wild rabbits to the surgery that when myxomatosis was suspected I intended to put the animal to sleep. Most people who lived nearby and enjoyed the countryside had seen rabbits in the late stages of the disease. Some of the bodies of affected rabbits are so disfigured as a result of the infection that it is a shock to the dog's owner who go to investigate what their pet is so interested in. To make matters even gorier the carcass had often been attacked by carrion crows or torn apart by a fox, but fortunately it was more common for the fox to carry off all the evidence. It came as a shock to town-dwellers facing the disease for the first time; it could have been their first experience of epidemic disease in wildlife.

I can remember as a schoolboy reading the first reports of the disease, brought on by a virus, which I stress only causes illness in the rabbit family, but for them is deadly and highly contagious. The fascinating story of the French doctor who tried to use the disease to control the number of rabbits on his estate is a good illustration of just how contagious the virus is. In 1952 he imported the virus and released a few infected animals to mix with his local rabbits. He successfully destroyed all the rabbits on his estate, but, within eighteen months, he had also managed to wipe out most of the rabbits in France, Germany, Belgium and Holland. It soon crossed the Channel and the disease established itself in England; the first cases were found in Kent in 1953. Attempts were made to eradicate the disease but it spread rapidly through the country, and an estimated 60 million rabbits died in the first epidemic. Nevertheless, some rabbits did recover and became immune to further infection, went on to breed and passed on their immunity to their offspring.

The infection can be passed from one animal to another by close contact but usually the virus is transmitted by the bite of an infected rabbit flea. The characteristic signs of the illness begin to develop about a week later, when the head and eyelids swell rapidly, and they have difficulty seeing through inflamed purulent eyes. Tumour lumps start to grow on the body. It is a horrific sight, but strangely they can sometimes be found feeding until just a few hours before they die. There is no specific treatment and, if a 'myxy' rabbit is found, speedy humane euthanasia is the only sensible course of action. Despite the horrendous effect the virus has on rabbits, hares are generally immune, and the virus will not cause illness in any domestic animals – apart from the pet bunny of course – and these really should be vaccinated each year against myxomatosis for peace of mind. The vaccine will not always give complete protection to these pets but should the vaccinated rabbit get infected it does improve their chances of being nursed back to health. It is not uncommon for the family cat, to the horror of the owner, to bring home a present of a young myxy rabbit by way of a change from a mouse, but he will never catch the disease. And dogs will be dogs and by the time the owner catches up with him the initial interest in the carcass might have progressed to sampling it. It looks disgusting but he will never get the disease either. I have lost count of how many times I have enjoyed that reassuring chat on the telephone with terrified owners.

Over the years our knowledge of the medical problems of the guinea pig, the mouse, the gerbil and all the other small rodents that children love to keep as pets grew steadily. The scant information we started out with in the 1960s had become volumes of expert advice by the time I retired.

Operative surgery using sophisticated controlled anaesthesia has become a routine procedure. The accurately weighed patient is given a combination of carefully calculated sedative drugs and at the appropriate time put into an anaesthetic chamber into which a controlled amount of gaseous anaesthetic is introduced. Within minutes the animal gently passes into a state of safe general anaesthesia.

How different it was in the 1960s. The pet with the fractured limb still needed a general anaesthetic to apply a Plaster of Paris cast in the case of the larger pets, or possibly a sticky Elastoplast tape bandage in the case of smaller ones. It was surprising how well fractured bones healed after the limb had been immobilised for a couple of weeks. How I was going to deal with that hamster with the overgrown teeth was something I might have thought about whilst out calving a cow. Most of us vets would have preferred to have continued calving cows all day. Who could possibly be worried about that hamster with the overgrown tooth? Well, the first problem could be a social one. More often than not the animal was the pet of Lady Fitzgerald's niece who assumed that the outcome of the operation would be a success. You dared not think about the consequences of a disastrous one. The second problem was a practical one: administering a general anaesthetic. Veterinary science had moved on from using a jam jar with ether on a ball of cotton wool. Now we were using the gaseous machine to administer general anaesthetics to dogs and cats, with a face-mask that had been designed for use on human infants. It was the tiniest available and I am sure it worked well with babies, but gerbils and hamsters were quite clever at escaping from your grip and disappearing up the mask. Putting your hand in to retrieve the patient was just one of the many painful times we vets discovered how uncooperative the hamster can be. Suddenly those overgrown incisor teeth that were preventing him eating his food are making a meal of your hand. With his teeth embedded in your fingers he has no intention of releasing his grip. A flick of the hand – accompanied by an expletive – normally does the trick, but there were occasions when it can result in the patient being propelled unceremoniously across the room, to the astonishment of the assisting nurse.

The pet always seemed to survive the ordeal and the vet, with blood still oozing from a deep finger wound, reapplies the mask, this time ensuring a tighter grip. There was always the risk of a bite occurring during a consultation with the owners. Naturally no vet in their right mind would deliberately throw their patient against the consulting room wall, or issue profanities for the entire neighbourhood to hear, but it has been known. Such was the case in the '70s when the owners of a small rodent were not convinced of the vet's good intentions and refused to accept his explanation. Following a complaint, the unfortunate vet was hauled up before the Royal College's Disciplinary Committee. There he was found to have acted in an unprofessional manner and was struck off. For practising vets at that time, it was difficult to understand how the committee members could have come to this decision. Clearly they had never experienced a hamster hanging on to their bleeding finger. Perhaps on those traumatic occasions when they stood up and bashed their heads on the shelf above they complained, 'Oh silly me, what a foolish thing to do, I must try to be more careful in the future.' It is only natural for a vet to utter something sharp and spontaneous immediately following a kick, scratch or bite, and then apologise to anyone present. An experienced nurse learns to ignore such language on these occassions.

Looking back on what could have happened when dealing with exotic creatures, I think I was fortunate to survive relatively unscathed. An occasion that could have left me permanently marked occurred whilst routinely treating a lizard for worms. I was expecting the creature to arrive at some stage during the evening: I had overheard the nurse arranging the appointment. I looked forward to him arriving; treating a lizard made an interesting change from the routine of vaccinating and clipping nails, and of course the emptying of anal glands. I recall searching the Gloucestershire countryside and exploring disused Cotswold stone quarries as a boy for small, friendly harmless lizards. I was not too sure about this particular monitor lizard when he arrived. He was huge. At first glance you could have been excused for thinking it was a baby alligator. The owner placed him on the examination table and I reassessed the amount of liquid anthelmintic I had planned to administer.

I approached my patient. He continued to look straight ahead as I approached him from the side with a small standard 2ml syringe, filled with a white suspension of Panacur. This was an effective and reliable drug that was safe to give to most creatures. It was my intention to gently introduce the syringe into his mouth and squeeze the plunger.

He saw me coming faster than I saw him move. It was astonishing, the syringe simply shattered as he spun round and snapped at it. I cannot remember what I said at that time but fortunately the owners were understanding and happy at my suggestion that perhaps it would be wiser to dispense with the direct anthelmintic approach and administer something in his food.

Today, veterinary practitioners are fortunate that in the same way that their medical counterparts are able to refer patients to a consultant specialist, they are able to do likewise. Just a decade ago the second opinion consultants were few and far between. Consequently, the local vet often relied upon his ingenuity to overcome a medical problem.

Not long after the monitor lizard incident, another exotic reptile was presented at surgery. He was a big iguana that originated from Down Hatherley. He had travelled just a few miles to see us with his necrotic scorched tail, which had become gangrenous and infected. To his detriment he had managed to get too close to the hot lamps keeping him warm in his vivarium and been seriously burnt. To save his life it was necessary to remove the lifeless necrotic appendage – in other words his tail had to come off. After a brief refresher on reptilian anatomy I was confident that the surgery would present no unexpected problems. My main concern was administering that general anaesthetic.

Coincidentally, just a few days before, I had been reading of a challenge presented by Arnolds, the old British established veterinary instrument company. At this time they were manufacturing innovative plastic products as well as their beautiful stainless steel instruments.

'What uses can you make of our plastic urinary catheters?' Arnolds asked. 'Well, for a start', I said to myself, 'I think the smallest size would fit comfortably into the trachea of an iguana awaiting surgery and it could be a totally suitable endotracheal tube.' As it turned out, it was a perfect fit and worked a treat. Two weeks later the sutures had been removed and the patient was making a speedy recovery. My nurse and I had enjoyed performing the operation. At that time it was unique, we thought, and we were pleased with the outcome. My nurse had taken pictures during the procedure and I was happy for her to forward an account of the operation to Arnolds and to submit it as an entry in their national competition. And guess what? We won!

Over the years life with exotic pets in the practice was fun and led to many stories that have been related time and again to friends. I have written of just a few of them here. I had the interest but not the time in which to specialise in these weird and wonderful animals and I accepted my limitations.

To this day I recall with some amusement a consultation one Sunday morning with two local youngsters. They presented a glass jar that was thick with foliage and a variety of vegetation in the midst of which, they claimed, were their pet stick insects. It was a routine health check to assure them that they were doing all that was required to maintain the optimum health of their pets. To be honest I could not see anything in that jar other than the foliage. There were two possibilities: either their feeding and management was excellent, and resulted in the insects maintaining a complete natural camouflage, or they had knowingly presented an empty jar and were testing the limits of my professional vocabulary. I gave them the benefit of the doubt, complimented them on their excellent pet keeping and told them to keep up the good work. I was over the moon when they didn't ask me to sex them.

There was the odd occasion when my unprofessional vocabulary was tested to the limit. For many years at the start of surgery every Monday evening, the same woman came in with her undisciplined Jack Russell dog and her two unruly children. The girl was not too bad but the boy was something else. After just a twenty-minute session with them on a good night, they left my consulting room, went to reception and made an appointment for the following Monday evening. A typical consultation began with an account of everything the dog, Snoopy, had eaten that week and a weight check to ensure he had not gained or lost the odd ounce. I blamed any deviation on the faulty scales to avoid the owner panicking over any apparent change in the last seven days. Nevertheless it was only minutes before the conversation started on diets, adequate vitamin intake, water consumption and the condition of his coat. I confirmed each week that he required no vaccinations for at least four months and, as we had only wormed him the week before last, he required no more pills at the moment. Naturally I had to inspect his teeth, avoiding a bite, and muzzle him while I clipped his nails, and, if he had not already squirted his anal glands over the table or my arm, I emptied them as well.

While all this was going on I had to keep one eye on young Johnny. His favourite sport was belting around my room on the anaesthetic trolley. Then he would empty my cupboards and drawers of bandages, cotton wool, Elastoplast, bottles of disinfectant and everything else a vet needs to do his job. I could have made good use of the calving ropes but I wasn't allowed to tie him up. One Monday, after dismantling everything, he tried a new trick and started playing with the pneumatic pedal that adjusted the height of the operating table. He forgot that he had lowered it and when his mother told him to get out because they were leaving he stood up and hit his head on the solid metal underside of the table. He bawled his head off and, with great difficulty, I managed to keep a straight face and refrained from saying, 'Got you at last.'

'It serves you right', his mother shouted, louder than he was yelling. 'I keep telling you to behave yourself at the vets.'

CHAPTER TEN

IN SICKNESS AND
IN HEALTH

From a very early age it was clear to me that one of the most important things in life was good health. I thanked my lucky stars that by hook or by crook I overcame the early setbacks that I had experienced as a child and went on to enjoy what was essentially a fit and happy life.

I had learned, perhaps subconsciously, that no matter how much wealth you accumulated in life, contentment, happiness, respect and the company of true friends were things you could not buy. Having said that, the health and fitness ideal was often a struggle for this particular veterinary practitioner to maintain, particularly when his patients were determined to prove otherwise. Frequently, at the end of the day, I eased my sore body into bed and refused to count sheep to get to sleep. I had seen too many of them.

The mental picture of the lad in the back row in the schoolroom wearing his baseball cap would have appeared in my mind. 'Have you ever been bitten, Mister?' He could also have enquired about being kicked, scratched, trampled, gored, stung or punched, to add a few of the occasional indignities. I could have replied in the affirmative to all of the above but I did not want him to get too excited. Much more seriously, I probably played another aspect of my professional life down as well: the constant exposure to infectious organisms that caused illness and death in my patients and were ready to make life rather unpleasant for the vet too.

One of the biggest fears for the practising vet was the possibility of contracting anthrax, and because it was not a rare disease, farm animals found dead without an obvious cause were tested for it. Because anthrax is officially a notifiable disease, the owner is required by law to report the sudden death to his vet, who then takes the necessary samples to examine in the practice laboratory. A smear of the animal's blood is carefully taken from a superficial ear vein on a glass slide and the specimen is stained with methylene blue. After further brief heat treatment the slide is ready to be examined under a microscope. At Vet School the stained appearance of the large microscopic encapsulated bacterium was drummed into us.

You hoped you would never see them and usually you did not, and having assured yourself and MAFF that the cow had not died from anthrax the carcass would be transported to the local knacker's yard. In our case it was usually to the local family firm of Ormond Eeles & Sons, of Longlevens. From schooldays until almost the time I retired, the boss was Walter Eeles. If you had the pleasure of meeting him it was difficult to believe that anyone else could possibly ever have been the boss. Walter ruled the Paygrove Lane establishment like a human Rottweiler, but as so often in such people, I believe he had a heart of gold. As a veterinary surgeon he treated me with the utmost respect, and I am sure other local vets experienced the same courtesy.

Nevertheless, I was careful never to remind him that as a 1960s teenage vet student studying first year anatomy at Liverpool I had, with a little trepidation, one bright wintry Sunday morning requested a horse's head and other superfluous equine bits and pieces.

'What the bloody 'ell do you want those for?' he's asked. I managed to look him in the eye and almost recognised a suppressed grin. He knew darned well what I wanted them for. He told me to come back the next day and I did what I was told (just like everyone else there I imagine). By then the selected bits of skeleton had been boiled in order to remove the soft tissues and to sterilise the bones, and they were ready for me to collect. I left Walter's yard on my bike with a sack on my back containing a horse's skull, and other large bones of significance.

To the local veterinary surgeons who at the time were mainly involved in large animal farm practice, and that was most of us, Walter was worth his weight in gold. As the years went by his weight in gold became quite substantial, but his deftness with a knife and ability to expose the viscera of a horse, cow or sheep – and probably anything else brought to his yard – was quite remarkable. Within minutes we often found ourselves discussing the post-mortem pathology of equine hearts and bovine livers, which had been a clinical enigma in life.

Walter called a spade a spade more frequently and vehemently than any north countryman I have ever met, though often with good reason. There was one occasion when a cow suffering a sudden death had escaped the diagnostic net and the carcass appeared in Walter's yard for routine butchering. Walter sliced open the cow's abdomen and a gigantic diagnostic spleen rolled on to the floor in front of him. I suspect that this was not the first time he had observed one of these because, on good authority I am assured, his immediate response, 'It's friggin' anthrax!', was bellowed loudly enough to ensure that everyone within half a mile understood the seriousness of the situation.

It was no surprise that Walter's diagnosis was correct but official confirmation was needed and within minutes of a telephone call to MAFF and the Veterinary Investigation Centre at Elmbridge Court, a mile or so away, a Ministry vet arrived and took the appropriate pathology samples. Within the hour Walter's yard had been officially declared an Infected Premises, complete with all the legislation that went with it. He was not too pleased with the inconvenience and did not take kindly either to the newspaper reports that naturally followed. He did after all provide hundreds of owners of carnivorous pets with a very economical and nutritious supply of meat. In theory, it was just possible that if any anthrax-contaminated foodstuffs were fed to the pets they too could become infected, and he was not amused by the adverse publicity. This was another occassion where he did not mince his words!

By coincidence at that time a worried lady brought her very dejected Lurcher type of dog to surgery. He had not been well for several days, but other than being 'off colour' he had shown no particular signs of ill-health. I lifted him gently on to my consultation table and began my routine examination. I removed the thermometer from his rectum, wiped it with a swab of spirited cotton wool and read his temperature. The column of mercury seemed to be trying to escape at the other end. To check my findings I once more inserted the thermometer. My patient buckled before me, collapsed onto the table, and died. To add to my concerns, the owner had offered the information that she had been feeding him meat purchased from – well, you can guess where.

Still trying to make sense of what had taken place in the last few minutes, I decided that I should just check the dog as a possible anthrax case, aware that the chance of this was remote in the extreme. Minutes later, I stared unbelievably down my microscope at the large bacillary organisms in the blood sample I had taken from the dog. They were not dissimilar in appearance to anthrax organisms. I telephoned my veterinary colleagues at Elmbridge Court and explained my findings to the micro-biological experts. 'Bloomin 'eck', said the vet pathologist on the end of the line. 'Just lock your surgery door and get the slide down here as quick as you can.'

Unfortunately, I tried to get the samples to them too quickly, as I explained to the police officers who waved me down in Parton Road. I admitted I was doing more than 30mph but I was definitely doing less than 40mph. I was clocked somewhere in between. In the '70s the road was still a relatively quiet village road and I believed on this occasion there might be mitigating circumstances. The officer noted at length most of what I had told him and informed me that it was very interesting and the facts would be passed to the chief constable, who would decide whether or not to prosecute me.

The chief constable was clearly not an animal lover. I paid my fine and hoped the accountants would look upon it as an essential motoring expense. By lunchtime, and to my great relief, the Ministry vets had confirmed that the anthrax-like bacteria were another group of similar organisms and my surgery would not be officially designated an Infected Premises. I had had more than enough legislation for one day.

But what was the Lurcher's cause of death? I can only guess, but over the years I have thought a lot about this case. Within weeks, in our small part of the world we saw many cases of canine parvovirus disease, which was spreading rapidly across continents. This was possibly the first case I had encountered, and thank heavens it was a new disease that we humans could not catch. It would, however, be devastating to the dog world.

We did not need any new ones to add to the list of zoonotic diseases; there were already enough out there to cope with.

Probably the one of most concern to young vets going into farm practice in the 1960s was the realisation that you would never be far away from Brucella abortus infection. We were lectured at Vet School about the seriousness of the disease and the enormous economic loss it caused in dairy herds. The disease was suspected when several cows in the herd aborted their calves in late pregnancy. Many of the aborting animals needed obstetrical assistance and the later in the pregnancy the problem arose, the more difficult it often was to remove the unborn calf. It was not uncommon to spend an hour with your arm inside the patient's reproductive tract. We did our best to avoid direct contact with infection, but it was a hopeless task. The arm-length plastic gloves were just too thin, and dealing with a difficult case resulted in torn gloves within minutes. Then you knew that your skin was in direct contact with foetal fluids that were teeming with Brucella bacteria. At the end of the delivery we scrubbed and scrubbed our skin with soapy iodine-based disinfectants, and hoped for the best. This was probably the way most young vets were infected initially, but there were other routes.

Most cows, following a normal healthy calving, will part company with their foetal membranes quite soon after birth. Cattle that had aborted tended to hang on to the placenta for many days and frequently became ill. Once again you hoped the plastic glove would not split when you plunged your arm into the vaginal tract and the uterus and carefully removed the infected tissues that were often bathed in foul-smelling discharges. The odour remained with you for the rest of the day and it was astonishing how often this task was carried out just before it was time for lunch.

Unfortunately, no matter how careful you were in avoiding skin contact, it was possible to become infected by breathing infectious dusty particles from the rear of the cow. This source came to light when a couple of window cleaners at the government's Central Laboratory at Weighbridge, who had never been near a cow in their lives, became infected. A glass vessel containing Brucella material was accidentally broken and a small amount of the substance was drawn into the building's air conditioning system. The bacteria wafted into the room where the cleaners were working and, in due course, they developed the clinical signs of brucellosis. There was however a rough and ready way of reducing the risk of breathing in infected particles. The first thing to do before examining the cow was to throw a couple of buckets of hot soapy water and disinfectant over her rear end to lay the dust.

As if inhaling the bacteria was not enough, another frequent entry for Brucella bacteria was through digestion. From the first day we moved into Odd Farm in Crudwell we accepted our neighbours' generous offer of supplying us with delicious milk straight from the cow, and walking to the farm for a chat was a pleasant daily routine Angela enjoyed. But within weeks both of us were suffering from a type of flu-like illness that lasted for weeks. It was months before Brucella infection was identified in Stanley's dairy herd and probably by then we had both been infected by our fresh daily pints. Angela recovered from the illness within weeks and made a full recovery. It could have been much more serious, but fortunately she was not constantly exposed to the infection.

A worrying aspect of the situation at the time was the medical profession's apparent lack of awareness, certainly at local level, of the public health significance of Brucellosis. The prevalence of the infection did not seem to be recognised, even though in country practices doctors would have been surrounded by the disease. This was my experience and it was many years before I encountered a doctor who appreciated the importance of it. During the few days I spent in the small cottage hospital in Cirencester having my tonsillectomy I had the chance to strike up a friendly relationship with a newly qualified young doctor and enjoyed many chats with him between the very restricted visiting hours. He had indeed heard of human brucellosis, but he related this to a form of the illness known to medics as undulant fever, which was caused by Brucella melitensis. This was more likely contracted as a result of contact with infected goats in hot climates.

Strangely it was several years, despite almost daily exposure to the infection, before it began to cause me a serious health problem – no doubt I had developed some immunity to it. I was then living in Churchdown and had been involved in cattle practice for about ten years before the classic signs began to develop. I began to wake each morning with the characteristic muscular and joint pains and wishing I could spend the rest of the day in bed. Analgesic tablets were taken with my morning tea and off I went to surgery. By lunchtime the nurses were mopping the sweat from my face as we stood around the operating table, and I longed to sit down and take more analgesics. When the symptoms dragged into the third week I knew it was time for a trip to the doctor. As so often happens, you seem to find yourself improving the day you consult the doctor. I walked into Dr Jimmy Caldwell's room and explained that I was feeling much better.

'You don't look much better to me', he remarked. 'Sit down, and put this in your mouth.' He passed me a thermometer. He picked up his telephone and rang the Public Health Laboratory in Gloucester. Half an hour later the array of blood samples he had been asked to take were lined up in tubes on his desk. Jimmy telephoned me a few days later, and I am sure it came as no surprise to either of us that my antibody levels to the various brucellosis blood tests were sky high. Over the next couple of months, and following weeks of antibiotic treatment, the blood picture returned to normal and, touch wood, brucellosis has not troubled me since. I think today's aches and pains must be due to something else.

A few years later I became a bit concerned when another apparent bout of flu once more dragged into a third week. I began to think to myself, 'Oh dear, here we go again.' Jimmy took the required blood samples and we chatted about how rapidly things had improved over the years in the diagnosis of so many diseases in both the human and veterinary fields. Now the Public Health Laboratory had put together a diagnostic package where blood tests for numerous diseases were incorporated that were particularly relevant to vets, farmers and anyone else who worked with animals. It was interesting that as well as brucellosis being on the list, so too was psittacosis, the illness occasionally contracted from birds and caused by the bacteria chlamydia psittaci. While we joked about 'sick parrots', I happened to mention a mynah bird that I had treated some time back for a large painful conjunctival abscess, and thought no more of it until many weeks later. In many ways it was frustrating not to have shown an antibody response to any of the tests. I still felt very much under the weather.

'I think we'll do them again', Jimmy said. He was right; when the tests were completed on the second occasion the laboratory rang to tell us my blood titres to chlamydia psittaci infection were rocketing. I had psittacosis. I was back on the antibiotics for another couple of months. Occasionally this disease can lead to serious complications and I was relieved to find that the results of my ECG and chest X-rays showed that I had not suffered permanent heart or lung problems. These despondent recollections are rather gloomy. Let's move on quickly.

The skin infections transmitted from animals were a nuisance but not usually serious, and the most troublesome of the lot was ringworm. All species of animal have their own particular pathogens but most of these different fungi are happy to grow on human skin if the opportunity arises. Ringworm is a very common skin disease of cattle, particularly in young stock, and not surprisingly there is often a heavy level of infection in buildings where they are reared. In my early days in practice I quite enjoyed the daily sessions of disbudding calves or in the case of the older animals, where the farmer had not got round to arranging the job, removing the horns by sawing them off. In either case the calves had to be caught, and restraining the larger animals was as close as I came to playing a game of rugby at that time. Having lassoed the liveliest of the animals it usually took another couple of circuits of the barn before he was outnumbered and gave up further resistance. On one occasion I had a calf in an armlock when my wrist – in contact with a Cotswold-stone wall – was pulled rapidly forward, resulting in a deep skin abrasion to the back of my wrist. The wound appeared to heal satisfactorily and the pruritus I believed was part of the natural healing process, until the enormous scab lifted a few weeks later. Beneath it was a classical textbook ringworm lesion. This took longer to clear up than the original wound. Whitefield ointment prescribed by my doctor was applied daily, and I am sure this ancient application would be a useful remedy today if still available.

Ringworm is less common in smaller animals but common enough to be diagnosed frequently in the surgery. Cats are usually the patients brought in with skin changes that are sometimes scabby eczematous circumscribed lesions but may be little more than a dull coat and a few broken hairs to suggest that the fungal infection is present. Most cat owners have very close contact with their pet, and if ringworm was suspected the question was routinely asked, 'Do any members of the family have any unusual skin lesions?' It was always a good diagnostic question to ask and often resulted in advising the owner to have a chat with their doctor.

Traditionally vets, until quite recent times, wore smartly pressed white smocks in the consulting room, which I am sure impressed the client, certainly at the beginning of the surgery. Any stain on your uniform stood out like a sore thumb so on a bad day you could get through two or three coats. It was common practice for doctors to wear similar white coats at that time and an embarrassing situation occasionally arose when owners got carried away during the consultation and forgot that they were addressing the animal's doctor. It was amazing to hear the owner ramble on about their own ailments before I could remind them of my professional, social and legal limitations.

I suspected that Mrs Higginbottom's cat had ringworm when she placed him gently on my examination table. I asked the usual questions, including the one relating to a possible family skin problem.

'Yes, there is! It's all over me. I'm covered in it', she proclaimed, unbuttoning her blouse.

'It's all up my legs' she affirmed, lifting her skirt. All I need now, I thought, was for a nurse to walk in – and I have no idea how I am going to explain away this one. I rapidly assured my client that I had seen enough and pointed her in the direction of the doctors' surgery. I hoped that she wouldn't simply ask them to confirm the vet's diagnosis.

I think my main concern was going down with flu. It was impossible to avoid the virus when the ailing pet owner brought an animal to surgery and, for ten minutes or more while the examination took place, we shared the same air space.

Rotten colds we could cope with, but flu was a challenge we could do without, particularly in the early days of the practice when we were trying to maintain a twenty-four hour service single handed. We used to joke about the diagnostic test to distinguish between a bad cold and flu. If you came across a £5 note on the pavement and you were suffering from a cold you would bend down and pick it up. If you had flu you would leave it where it was. There were two or three occasions when I would have been happy to have left it there. Turning out to calve a cow on a winter's night, hoping the Beecham's Powder would soon kick in, was one thing. Failing to calve the cow, and spending the following couple of hours doing a bovine caesarean operation, is something which I am pleased to have few memories.

There were of course many more infectious diseases that we were always aware of. We did our best to avoid them and generally we succeeded.

What we were not quite so clever at from time to time was avoiding physical assaults from our patients. Surprisingly, we were rarely bitten by the Rottweiler. We were occasionally, but the villain was more likely a Jack Russell or one of his terrier friends.

A vet in practice quickly develops a sixth sense regarding a possible or impending attack. You simply do not push your luck with a large aggressive dog. That is what the strong leather muzzle was designed for. Experience taught you to get that muzzle on before the handsome, unpredictable golden retriever got his retaliation in first, and the apparently surprised owner exclaimed, 'I've never seen him do that before!' We tried to remain polite and just muttered to ourselves, 'Pull the other one.'

The occasional serious bite usually came out of the blue, and a bad one occurred on Saturday 5 November 1973. Morning surgery had been uneventful until my receptionist quietly mentioned that she had received a call on behalf of a couple whose neighbour was on his way to the surgery to have their dog put to sleep. It sounded rather dramatic. Apparently the owners had been taken to hospital with serious facial injuries caused by their pet dog and the neighbour had been delegated the job of sorting out the veterinary side. It had been customary on a Saturday morning for the husband to take his wife a cup of tea to the bedroom. For whatever reason on this particular morning the dog took exception to this, dived on to the bed, ignored the crockery and began to attack the wife, starting with her face. Naturally the husband went to her defence and he too was badly savaged. Both of them left in the ambulance.

When the shaking neighbour arrived at surgery we assured him that we fully understood the circumstances and would do what was necessary. It was shortly after that he unwisely released the lead from the dog's collar. Now we were alone in the consulting room, two strangers and a poor demented dog who wanted to attack everyone. I had met the dog previously but on this occasion, no matter how reassuring I had been to him in the past, now it meant nothing. I tried to speak to him quietly and did manage to get a hand to his head and stroked it gently. There was some response but his mind was in complete confusion. I grasped his collar, introduced the sharp needle under the skin of his neck and injected a very powerful sedative. He would have felt nothing from the injection, but he responded to my tightening grip on his collar, which to my dismay was too slack to control him. He squirmed and twisted and turned. Within seconds he had rolled over and now his jaws were in contact with my arm and his teeth were tearing into my wrist.

I could tell immediately that this was not an ordinary bite, and needed to know quickly how much damage had been inflicted. The unfortunate neighbour had been forced to watch the tussle and, as I looked up from the canine, I realised that I may soon have another patient requiring treatment. He said something like, 'Oh God, did he get you?' I probably replied, 'Yes, but it's nothing to worry about', and hoped he would quickly leave. I remember the next lines clearly.

'I think you've got a nasty bite there, son, let me have a look at it.' As I lifted my arm and exposed the wound at the end of the sleeve of my white coat the jagged margins of the lacerated skin parted and revealed quite a remarkable dissection. Every artery, vein, nerve and tendon sheath in that region seemed to be on display. Some of the tendons looked a little frayed to me as well. Perhaps they did to the neighbour too. He suddenly turned paler and buckled at the knees. Now there were three of us in the room in varying degrees of being a bit under the weather. I'm sure, as he lay on the floor next to his neighbour's dog, that he hadn't reckoned on something like this happening when he offered to take the dog to the vet this morning. A rough and ready sterile bandage sufficed until the end of morning surgery, when my veterinary nurse cleaned the wound in the iodine-based Pevidene, applied a sterile gauze that was impregnated with antibiotic, applied a soft dressing to protect the injury, secured it with a gauze bandage and finally applied our secret weapon: a long strip of narrow-width sticky Elastoplast tape. The latter usually outwitted most of our patients' attempts to remove a dressing.

As she wrapped the tape snugly around the hairs on my wrist, I am sure my nurse was experiencing a secret delight, taking pleasure in foreseeing someone else taking it off roughly. She rang our local doctor's surgery, explained what had happened, and they suggested I went along to see the doctor as soon as I could. When the elderly doctor on duty that morning removed the dressings from my arm his first words were, 'Where did you get these from?' before discarding them. I explained what and who and when, and the conversation mellowed. He changed his spectacles and looked inquisitively at my wound, took interest in the tendons and tweaked at the fragments with forceps that I hoped were straight out of the steriliser.

'It's obviously quite painful', he said sympathetically. I agreed. 'I think you may have some nerve damage, so perhaps I should send you to the Casualty Department in Gloucester.'

'Do you think so?' I replied, knowing full well that I would not be seeing a neuro-surgeon by chance on a Saturday morning.

'Perhaps not then', he agreed. 'I'll put a dressing on the wound and I suggest you make an appointment to see Dr Caldwell on Monday morning.'

We were in full agreement again and the doctor produced his bandages. He started to cover his dry dressing with what seemed like yards of cotton bandage that he struggled to remove from its cellophane wrappings. When he accidentally dropped the bandage roll, it sped across his surgery floor, unravelling as it went. The doctor got down on his hands and knees to pick it up, spent ages rewinding it, and then unwinding it back onto me. I eventually managed to politely escape and thanked the kind old doctor for his efforts. By Monday I was well on the mend and while relating the events of the weekend, Jimmy and I enjoyed a few professional wry smiles.

When I left the doctor's surgery I suspected it would not be too long before one of our veterinary practice members would be back for treatment. It was not very long and, going out of turn, it was me again. At the end of morning surgery a few weeks later, I quickly swallowed a tepid cup of coffee that the nurses had made half an hour before, heaped a pile of dressings into the car, and sped off to visit a bay mare that I had seen on several occasions over the last couple of weeks. She had suffered an extensive shin wound – the result of a kick from another horse – and had been very cooperative when I had dressed the leg and given injections of antibiotics and tetanus vaccine at the time of the injury.

I had been to the small riding centre and given more injections over the following few days. Even without the presence of the lady owner I had been quite happy to examine the mare in her stable without any assistance, and she had stood quietly as I firmly patted her neck, inserted the needle on the third pat and attached the syringe. She hardly flinched as the large volume of antibiotic entered her neck muscles. She seemed so trusting and well-behaved that I could never have imagined what was to follow.

I pulled into the yard and was greeted by the friendly smile of the owner. Her mare looked well and was clearly recovering from the injury she had sustained. Before giving her the all-clear, I wanted to check her out fully and to do this the rugs she was wearing needed to be removed. The owner began to unbuckle her while I stood in the safe area in front of her left hind leg, the position where in theory, because a horse cannot kick forwards, you are assumed to be safe.

What I did not know was that this horse had a serious vice. She panicked when rugs were removed. She bucked once and, before I knew it, she was in front of me and I was behind her – in the firing line. Then she let me have it. Her first kick caught me in the abdomen, and I had never experienced anything like it before. She put me into the air and kicked out a second time. This time she caught me in the chest and turned me over. To a spectator it must have looked like a circus act as I somersaulted and landed yards away on a woodpile. I tried to stand up but then fell back onto the logs as my legs gave way. I truly believed that the first time she kicked me her foot was inside me and it was the end of the road.

I eventually recovered enough to get back into my car and somehow drive back to Churchdown. I turned off Pirton Lane into St John's Avenue and pulled up outside the doctor's surgery. It was a little embarrassing slowly hobbling into the reception area, but it was reassuring to know that I was in good hands. There was no doctor available but the nurse's expert hands prodded me all over. Every diagnostic poke was followed by the question, 'Does that hurt?' I am sure I must have answered 'yes' to every one. My entire body hurt, but her final words were reassuring. 'I think you will survive again on this occasion, Mr Smith.'

Our children were amused by the equine foot imprints on my torso that changed from red to blue to yellow over the following weeks. Unfortunately I did not take pictures but I wish now that I had. It would be satisfying to remind my wife that my waist and abdomen were once a few sizes smaller.

From time to time other members of my veterinary staff did take their turn and attended the St John's Avenue surgery at short notice. Every day there was a chance that one of us would suffer a nasty dog bite, but we generally worried far more about cat bites and scratches. The worst occasion I experienced once again came out of the blue.

Every day in the '70s my RANA nurse Rosemary and I gave general anaesthetics to several cats and carried out their routine spays and castrations, the neutering operations. Today we would normally administer a potent sedative pre-operatively to the feline patient, intubate and then connect the cat to the anaesthetic machine. Between thirty and forty years ago we may still have used the same reliable and safe gaseous anaesthetic, but back then it was probably administered through a small face-mask. This was the situation on the day Rosemary and I carried out a routine cat castration.

How many times have I tried to impress on ambitious youngsters that nothing in veterinary practice is routine? The powerful cat released himself from Rosemary's grasp and sprang at her. His front claws tore at her head while his canine teeth sunk deep into her face and neck. Every moment resulted in more scratches; it was becoming horrific. I gripped his scruff and secured his head, easing the cat from her, but the painful scratches continued. Each time a foot was released and an attempt made to release another, the cat lashed out and clawed again. I forced his neck ever further backwards away from her, fearing that a claw would find Rosemary's eyes. It was many minutes before I managed to finally release the cat from every attachment and her desperate cries stopped.

My nurse's appearance was horrific; blood oozed from a seemingly endless array of punctures and scratches on her neck and face. Rosemary was tough, but the nightmare experience had sent her into a state of shock and she was in urgent need of medical attention. Within minutes she was in my secretary's car en route to the St John's Avenue surgery, and then on to Gloucester's Royal Hostpital. As I expected, she was back in our own surgery the following morning. She took antibiotics with her coffee for the next two weeks, and needless to say she made a rapid recovery. No doubt if I asked her today if she remembered the incident she would reply, 'You bet, I still have the scars to remind me.'

'Always expect the unexpected' was good advice to reduce the risk of being injured by your patients and only occasionally did I stray from it. From time to time I was reminded that there was no room for complacency. A painful reminder happened at the end of an evening session. This was often the time of day when owners arranged to bring their pets to the surgery for the last time so that they could be put to sleep. I believe it was a well-considered and understandable arrangement to avoid other owners and perhaps to postpone the distressing occasion for just a few hours longer. I fully understood those feelings.

This particular evening was a little different. The young Border Collie that arrived with his emotional owners was there as a result of having seriously bitten various members of the family and friends. From discussions I had had with the owners it was clearly a no-hope situation and I had agreed to carry out the euthanasia. They decided not to stay while I did the necessary and left my consultation room in tears. Although he had been brought to surgery muzzled, he had always seemed a nice dog to me and I had never been threatened by him on the several previous occasions I had examined him. We shaved his arm with the electric clippers, and my nurse swabbed the injection site. She raised the vein and I injected the barbiturate overdose painlessly into the prominent vessel. His tense body began to relax, and, in a moment of unwise sentiment, I removed his leather muzzle and stroked his head. The opportunity to have one last bite was too much. He snapped at my outstretched hand, connected, drew blood, and expired.

In my forty years in practice I have had my fair share of retaliation from my patients. I have never experienced physical violence or injury from any client and neither has my staff. I mention it because in this new violent world of ours it has become an occasional problem in veterinary practice and alarmingly a regular occurrence with our medical colleagues. Has my life ever been threatened? I hope only with tongue in cheek.

Overnight our profession became aware of the world of compensation and litigation-minded clients, and, every time someone left their animal at my surgery for a procedure that varied from extensive abdominal surgery to simply taking blood samples, they were asked to sign a disclaimer form. One lady who owned numerous pets that I had treated over the years was asked to sign the form for the first time.

'Why do I need to sign this?' she asked quite reasonably.

'Well, in case anything goes wrong, it means you won't be able to sue the practice.' It was blunt but true, and if you have read any of the previous chapters in this book then you can guess which honest, straight-to-the-point nurse said it. But surely it's better to come right out with the facts rather than have a client discover it hidden away in the small print at a later date? My trusting client replied, 'I don't need to sign that. If anything goes wrong I won't be suing him, I'll kill him.'

Decades on, we are still very good friends.

CHAPTER ELEVEN

CRIMINAL COTSWOLDS

Crime must seem an odd topic for someone whose career has revolved around the relatively peaceful world of animals, but strangely, by the end of some days, there was often reason to believe that not everything that day had been fair and square. The reason of course was that animals had owners, most of them anyway, and the vast majority were kind, responsible people who appreciated all that my practice did to help them and their animal families. It was the odd unappreciative, rude and unkind individual that made you feel you were losing faith in human nature. Strangely it was not particularly society's rogues who made me despondent. They seemed to live on their wits, diddled everyone, and frankly they occasionally brought a smile to our faces.

In an account reflecting on a lifetime of experiences in practice an occasional association with a villain was unavoidable. Many of these encounters produced unforgettable stories, some sad, some happy and some just plain unbelievable. Perhaps there is a little degree of criminality in many, perhaps all, of us but at least my clients had the reassurance that they had the support of the Royal College of Veterinary Surgeons' Disciplinary Committee to help keep their vet on the straight and narrow. A chastisement and a warning from a local magistrate to a vet for a particular misdemeanour, from a driving offence to a punch-up, might well be followed by an appearance before the DC, and the vet found guilty of unprofessional or disgraceful conduct and no longer worthy to practice, until they said so. That could be a very expensive secondary judgement.

Public honesty was seriously put to the test the day a lady from nearby Longlevens brought a magnificent and very expensive Amazon grey parrot into surgery. He had almost certainly escaped from a local home and was weak enough, probably from exhaustion, for the public-spirited lady to have picked him up and brought him to us. There were no signs of external injuries, but we admitted the beautiful bird and put him into a hospital cage where we could keep an eye on him. He recovered quickly without treatment other than food, water and nurses' TLC. He was comfortable in their hands but nevertheless, he was no doubt anxious to be reunited with his owners.

The local press provided a useful means to achieving this. They were normally very willing to come along and take a picture of a pet, usually in the arms of a veterinary nurse, and reported the story based on the details we provided. In this instance the Gloucester *Citizen* was as obliging as usual, and on the bird's second evening's stay, a nurse and the parrot had their moment of fame. It was an eye-catching picture and quickly spotted by a Longlevens reader who could not believe their good fortune. At about 4 p.m., at the start of surgery, one of my nurses popped into my room wearing her usual big smile to tell me the grateful owners of the parrot were on their way to collect their missing Amazon grey.

Less than an hour later the same nurse, this time without her smile, came into my room to say: 'I think we may have a problem, Mr Smith.'

'We have, Jane? What makes you think so?'

'Well, someone else has just phoned to tell us the parrot is theirs, but I've already given it to the first people who rang.'

Things were rapidly becoming a first-come-first-served situation, and we could have done with a few more parrots. Surgery ended at 7 p.m. and by then we had a list of five other callers who, by chance, had lost a £400 Amazon grey parrot that week. The duty vet diverted the practice telephone to his home. The eighth claimant rang shortly after he arrived, and it did not stop there. By the folowing morning we had a list of twenty-odd people in the Gloucester area, all of whom had lost a parrot. It needed the wisdom of Solomon to sort that one out.

The majority of our clients happily paid our professional fees and sincerely thanked us for our efforts. Farmers inevitably moaned about the fees but the majority of them paid their bills reasonably promptly. Some farmers just moaned about the fees and paid them slowly. It was unusual for a farmer not to moan and not to settle an account eventually. Naturally, as in all other walks of life, there was the one that never stopped complaining, was determined not to pay, and took his business elsewhere, where the cycle was repeated at a neighbouring veterinary practice.

The companion side of the practice was a little different with regard to finances and normally the pet owner was expected to settle the account on the completion of treatment, and this arrangement usually worked well. Nevertheless, between 5 and 10 per cent of the practice turnover could be written off every year in unpaid fees. Not all of it was the result of dishonesty.

Some related to the treatment of pets where their owners had hardly two pennies to rub together. Whether they should have taken on the animals in the first place is another matter. Often we found ourselves treating their pets regardless. It was sometimes possible to direct them to the RSPCA or one of the other charitable clinics, which was an immense help to the animal and to the grateful genuinely hard-up owner. It did not resolve the problem of course of the cat that was knocked over in the middle of the night or the collapsed dog that had been vomiting for days and had to be seen on Saturday afternoon. The situation was frustrating but I was convinced the only way to come to terms with the problem was to grin and bear it. It was arguably business madness but for me it was probably the only and right way of approaching an insoluble problem. It was less worrying to do what needed to be done now and argue about who paid for what later.

I was lucky enough to be present when one of the greatest veterinary surgeons of all time, Professor John George Wright, gave his swansong lecture to the Liverpool Vet School, and in his lengthy talk he referred to this matter. He reminded us that we were particularly fortunate individuals who were entering a profession where our livelihoods were protected by law. In a nutshell, the Veterinary Surgeons Act prevented anyone other than a registered vet from practising veterinary surgery. It was illegal for any other person to diagnose and treat the animals of others. As a consequence of this privilege he reminded us that we were obliged to attend the animals at any time we were asked. No one else could.

I resisted becoming too philanthropic, and my secretary reminded us all frequently that we were not running a charity. To be honest there were times when it was difficult to believe you were not becoming a cynic. We rapidly became wary of the owner who proclaimed at the first consultation, 'I want the animal put right. I don't care how much it costs.' He might well have added, 'Whatever it costs I don't intend paying anything anyway'. The Small Claims Court was a useful tool for retrieving some of the fees, but many of the outstanding debts were too small to make it worth while chasing them through the legal system. Over the years I lost just one case, and on that occasion we had made a clerical error in submitting our details to the court.

That particular day had not started well. The owner I was suing lived on a houseboat on the River Severn, and his attire was in keeping with a casual life on the river. His long black hair extended to his shoulders. His frayed denim jeans were supported by a very wide leather belt adorned with a huge brass buckle. An enormous sheath knife dangled from it. Somehow he had managed to obtain a green T-shirt with a slogan that read 'Royal Veterinary College Trust Fund'. Dressed in my grey suit and carrying my briefcase I followed him into the courtroom. We sat in front of the judge, whose first words were, 'Now then, which one of you is the vet?'

Going to court was often an expensive waste of time. Having won the case it was common for neither our professional fees nor the court fees to be paid and it usually meant that I would be away from the practice for at least half a day. Dishonesty seemed to be such a common trait that there were times when you began to wonder if it was part of being normal. I suppose if our political leaders often get away with fiddling the books and indulging in hanky panky on a scale that beggars belief, the man in the street has good reason to believe his lesser misdemeanours will be considered of little importance. The degree of criminality I experienced varied right across the board from one extreme to the other. I could not have been more unaware of one end of the spectrum that I was about to encounter one evening.

The telephone rang and a concerned owner described the suffering his dog was under as a result of what sounded like an acute ear infection. The problem needed speedy attention and, as he had no means of getting to the surgery, he asked if I would mind visiting him at his home in Brockworth. His Springer Spaniel was well behaved and there was no difficulty in gently inserting the speculum of the otoscope into the ear canal of the dejected patient, painful as it was. I gave a combination of antibiotic and analgesic injections, arranged to visit the next day, patted the patient's head and bade them good night. The dog barked and greeted me at the door on my next visit. He was making a rapid recovery. I gave more injections and dispensed antibiotic tablets and an ear preparation from my case. I enjoyed a cup of tea with the owner and, having given instructions and advice on how to insert an oily lotion into a painful ear, departed.

I thought little more of what was a routine case until a few weeks later, when my secretary Joan informed me that the account remained unpaid. The wording in her bill reminders, in usual fashion, became stronger, and finally the 'pay up now or else' letter went out. Months had passed since the first one had been posted, but Joan's letter at last provoked a response. She suggested I had a word with the irate chap on the telephone. The next five minutes were spent confirming that he did indeed live at the address I had visited, but was not the owner of a dog. In fact he made it abundantly clear he had never owned a dog. The arguing continued. Then suddenly there was an abrupt silence at the other end.

'Oh my God', he stuttered, 'Perhaps you did see a dog here. We were away for six months and we let the house to someone.'

'Well can you tell me who it was I saw that night?' He gave me the name.

'How can I get in touch with him?'

'If you really want to', he said, 'you can write to him c/o Her Majesty's Prison, Broadmoor.'

There was silence while I digested this information. It came as quite a surprise that I had enjoyed a cup of tea with someone who had met two young women hitch hikers on the Oxfordshire bypass, then raped and strangled them both. He looked quite ordinary to me.

Fortunately, most of the villains I came across were not wicked in that sense, in my view anyway, simply bored and misguided idiots.

My father often said, 'They wouldn't have been doing that if they had done National Service.' I agreed with him. Just about every mature person in the UK I have ever met would have agreed with my him too, except the politicians of course.

Nevertheless, some young robbers wasted a great deal of our time and caused us a lot of unnecessary expense. Our Churchdown surgery was not immune to attempted burglaries. We experienced the occasional broken window, but it was not such an easy target with me living close by with our attentive dogs. Jimmy was not a huge dog but I would not have wanted to get on the wrong side of her when she was in a defensive mood.

Our surgery at Brockworth, unoccupied at night, was more vulnerable. For many years it faced the Flying Machine pub on the other side of the road, which sadly achieved some notoriety. The locals in the bar must have enjoyed the entertainment one evening, wondering if an episode of *Some Mothers Do 'Ave 'Em* was being filmed there. Frank Spencer could not have performed better than our local comedian.

The young man breaking into the surgery chose to go in through the roof. Once through, if he had veered to his left, within moments he would have been over the drug store and the cash area, although there was not enough there to have bought him more than a few pints. To provide a little security we regularly left the lights of the waiting room on throughout the night. The locked areas where the petty cash and mostly harmless drugs were kept were in darkness. Shortly before pub closing time the burglar made his move and broke through the ceiling plasterboard. He squeezed through the hole and dangled his feet into the room below. The disorientated nincompoop descended into the illuminated waiting room. The Flying Machine regulars could not believe their eyes, and needless to say he was arrested by the strong arm of the Brockworth residents.

Over the years the Flying Machine pub became an enigma. For a long time it was just the place where locals put the world to rights and the local girl met the boy of her dreams. Eventually there was to be a more sinister association when it became part of the drug culture. Dealing in the pub and the car park were allegedly regular nightly and, eventually, daily activities. From the surgery the view across the road into the pub rooms and its car park were quite close and unobstructed and it came as little surprise when the police asked if we would allow them to spend some time in the surgery for surveillance purposes. For a while it was quite amusing when at the end of evening surgery Joan wished the police officer good night and locked him in. She probably told him to keep a watchful eye on the petty cash and the chocolate biscuits as well.

About this time a young fellow brought his Doberman to our Churchdown surgery one Sunday morning and expressed concern about the dog's behaviour. The dog certainly was behaving strangely. He seemed to be falling asleep on his feet. He responded if you spoke to him or stimulated him in some way and then began to doze off once more. I could find nothing really of clinical significance when I examined him, and certainly there were no findings that gave me a reason to be over-concerned. Nevertheless, something was interfering with his central nervous system.

From time to time dogs, and cats too, will manage to find household remedies or more potent medicines that have been prescribed to members of the family, and try them, out of curiosity. This was a possibility although the owner ruled it out. Swallowing garden chemicals, herbicides, insecticides and rodent poisons were other possibilities, but again the owner did not think this was likely. One of the added bonuses of practising as a vet for a long time in a community is the opportunity to be part of it. It is amazing how much you come to know about folks, their personal lives and their families. I knew much of the background of this particular likeable young man, his lifestyle, and the company he kept.

It would not have come as a surprise to hear that pot smoking was rife at one of his Saturday night parties, but that was not the uppermost thing on my mind when I dispensed palliative medicines to his dog, and almost in passing mentioned I would take samples if he had not fully recovered when I saw him the next day. I had not fully appreciated at the time that I had just examined my first patient suffering from the effects of marijuana. This had not been a topic included in my Liverpool Vet School curriculum.

The worried owner was waiting for me with his dog in the car park when I arrived at surgery the next day. I had hardly got out of my car when he asked for a quiet word, and began to explain what had indeed happened on Saturday night. The reference to me taking samples had clearly alarmed him. I suspect there was an association in his mind between clinical samples and criminal evidence. A few minutes later, with the Doberman standing alert on my table, it was pleasing to find that my patient had made a complete recovery. They left the surgery with the young owner promising me for about the fifth time that he would never let this happen again. I really did believe him.

Lord, when is a crime not a crime? I am not sure what the Lord might judge, but I think it was borderline one evening in the '80s when someone was using the cottage extension of the practice telephone line for their personal pleasure. Actually I think that BT was half to blame.

For some reason they considered that it was a useful service and no doubt a very profitable one to provide an early evening chat-line for lonesome chaps returning home from their place of work. In reality, a spicy dialogue between the caller and a fantasy girl at the other end took place if you dialled the correct expensive number. At this time one of our neighbouring Pound Cottages – parts of which dated back to the sixteenth century and had once been part of Pound Farm – was occupied by a young professional gentleman with very good credentials. I hasten to add that at this time it was not a vet, but perhaps I should have queried then why my bachelor veterinary assistants did not return home at the end of the day suffering similar frustrations.

From the veterinary surgery our receptionist naturally telephoned frequently to speak to our clients, using the surgery line, about matters relating to their pets. It was possible for a client to use some form of 'ring back', and that was what receptionist Susan believed one evening when she lifted the telephone and put it to her ear. Susan was a mature family lady but could not believe what she was hearing. She was alarmed by the sounds of deep breathing and the moans and groans of someone in apparent need of urgent medical care. Before ringing for an ambulance she felt it was wise to ask me for a second opinion.

'Oh, Mr Smith', she gasped (it was becoming contagious), 'I think one of our clients is having an attack of something, I don't know who she is and she won't tell me where she is.'

Susan passed the telphone to me and I had to admit it was not the usual sort of conversation I had with my clients. There certainly was an abundance of puffing and panting. Later, at the end of surgery, I tactfully explained to Susan what I thought the matter might be about, and told her that I would have a quiet word with the gentleman in the cottage next door. As promised, I did have a chat with our tenant the following evening and I am not sure who was more embarrassed, but there were no repeat episodes as far as I am aware. I cannot recall asking Susan to confirm that, but I had no further complaints from anybody. I cannot remember either if I ever checked BT's charges for this amusing interlude. Our generosity knew no bounds, but it is all part of life's experiences in this funny old world I suppose.

At the end of the working day I was happy to go home, relax and enjoy a delicious supper my wife had prepared. Like most families we put our feet up for an hour or so, and both Angela and I enjoyed watching documentaries. A favourite for many years was the BBC's *Panorama*. One evening we spent an hour watching a *Panorama Special* and listening to a reporter describe the inadequate funding of Britain's police forces. To illustrate their point effectively, they had chosen the force policing the rural Cotswolds where, it was claimed, there were just two police cars to cover goodness knows how many square miles of our beautiful countryside. One car was on duty through the night and the whole of the enormous area was protected by just one car through the day. If the insurance companies were watching the programme they must have been tearing their hair out. The Cotswolds answer to Al Capone must have been rubbing his hands together as he saw the one police car a day accelerate into the distance. Naturally the programme progressed to the consequences of the inadequate protection.

An idyllic film of Bourton-on-the-Water was shown, one of our Cotswold gems and one of the last places on earth you would expect to experience robbery with violence.

No doubt the point being made was that if there had been *two* police cars a day available this offence might not have happened. Recently, the reporter stated, unbelievably, there had been a ram raid in the main street and many televisions had been stolen from an electrical shop. Worse was to come. Leaving the devastation of broken glass, the offenders spied the shop's illuminated signs, which by chance contained the letter 'E'. The bounders pinched that as well. Why on earth would anyone want to do that? *Panorama* was about to explain. Apparently, the reporter revealed, 'If you want to show that you are really with it, you go to your next disco/club/rave/knees-up with a big plastic 'E' dangling from a necklace.' 'E' is for Ecstasy.

It took me back to the Liverpool road signs and the red and white cones that appeared from nowhere on a Sunday morning in our university's halls of residence. Young men have an inborn desire to collect trophies on a Saturday night. 'It would be sensible', we were advised by our head warden, Professor Seabourne-Davies, 'if you returned them straight away to where you found them.' This assumed that anyone could recall where they had found them. The advice had come from a good source; the professor was one of the country's leading criminal lawyers at the time.

My next day in the practice began with a morning session at our Brockworth surgery. Even before I entered the building for my 10 o'clock cup of coffee, I was aware that something at the surgery was different. This morning I was not heading towards the 'VETERINARY SURGERY', but the 'V–T-RINARY SURG-RY'. Now wasn't that a coincidence, *Panorama*?

It was an interesting but for us expensive exercise and we hope the kids enjoyed their moment of glory. We replaced the attractive Perspex letters with stick-on ones that were guaranteed to be non-peelable, and we hoped that the BBC would not repeat the programme any time soon.

Most of us enjoy a good practical joke, but causing unnecessary expensive damage becomes vandalism and is no longer funny. My sense of humour was stretched to breaking point when I had to replace a wall on the corner of Green Street. I had bought one of the neighbouring ancient Pound Cottages at the beginning of the '80s, a time when it was still customary for the veterinary practice to provide free accommodation for the vet assistants.

An elderly lady walking along Green Street was surprised to watch a car perform an unusual manoeuvre in the road in order to face the wall. The vehicle then accelerated into it before reversing back on to the road. The old wall had been dented but stood firm. The demolition gang however was not to be beaten. The second shot was more successful, and the car ended up on the paved area for a moment, partly buried in debris, before reversing; the vandals then drove off in the battered vehicle. I bet it wasn't even their car. The police interviewed the old lady, the sole witness. Despite being in a state of shock, she gave the police as much information as she was able. The police then knew they were looking for a black saloon and three or possibly four youths.

For a week or two, while arrangements were made for a builder to restore it, a pile of stones remained outside the cottage where once there had been a fine wall. By the time a stonemason arrived to begin building there were no longer enough Cotswold stones to fill the gap so more had to be bought. There seemed to be a secondary market in the vandalism business. Apparently at night various people had been seen wheelbarrowing stones off for their own use. The old wall was probably being transformed into fireplaces and garden rockeries all over Brockworth. I was pleased to see the rebuilding job completed before the original wall disappeared completely.

If the occupants of the car on that occasion had injured themselves they could have expected little sympathy; they would have had only themselves to blame. I have similar feelings for the mean, anti-social person who on one occasion smashed the surgery reception window with a brick just sufficiently to reach through and take the 'Guide Dogs for the Blind' collection box. How badly he gashed his arm on the jagged glass I have no idea, but there was a great deal of blood to clean up with the fragments of broken glass the following morning.

Perhaps he got what he deserved, but shortly after, in another surgery-related crime, a youngster got a little more than he deserved. On this occasion the lad ended up in hospital fighting for his life in intensive care. One of my assistants was a vet named Steve Butterworth who lived in Pound Cottage in the late '80s. He rang our main Churchdown surgery early one morning to let us know he would be a little late for work. Actually he asked for a lift; his Astra had disappeared early that morning from his parking spot outside the cottage. Apparently Astras were notoriously easy to break into. The police contacted Steve to tell him where his car was, and it was not too far away. It was quite easy to find along the road between Brockworth and Churchdown: a large gap in the roadside hedge pointed to where the car had left the road, and then bounced and rolled before settling on its roof. A trail of veterinary bandages, white dressings, cotton wool, and boxes of medicines and syringes led to the battered car. The two youngsters involved in the theft were very seriously hurt and one of them had neck injuries, leaving him paralysed at the time of the crash. One hopes the damage to his spine was not permanent and that he eventually recovered.

Having a car stolen is a very strange feeling. The immediate reaction for me was one of disbelief and denial. When I discovered one morning at The Brambles that my car was not in the place I believed I had parked it the night before, I began to rack my brains, assuming for a few moments that I must surely have parked elsewhere. After a few minutes came the realisation and acceptance that it had been stolen. My beautiful new little Ford Escort turbo had been pinched. If there was still any doubt in my mind, it quickly disappeared as I reported the details to the police. Within the hour I was back on the telephone letting the police know that my car, or most of it, had been located. It was in one of the ancient quarries at Birdlip and had been found by a Cotswold Park warden. There were enough personal details still in the car for him to identify me as the owner.

'I think you should get here as soon as possible, Mr Smith', he instructed me over the phone. 'I'm afraid they've already taken the wheels and the front seats, and if you don't come and get it soon, it won't be long before others come along and take some more of it.' There was obviously a secondary market in the car-nicking business too.

From time to time we lost other cars by the same route and when my restored Escort disappeared for the second time it was never seen again. On that occasion it was a truly professional job and the Manchester police informed me that my car was now probably part of another car. I never really understood why the crooks go to the trouble of sawing cars in half and joining two different ones together but no doubt there are sound profitable reasons. To add insult to injury I last saw my favourite stethoscope in a plastic bag marked 'exhibit 136'. It had been retained by the police as evidence; I had started to lose property to the bad guys *and* the good guys.

A particular concern regarding those who steal or just break into vets' cars is the possibility of them getting their hands on dangerous drugs. This was a problem that could only occur during the daytime. At night anything of concern was removed and placed under lock and key in the surgery. Should anyone be silly enough to try sampling anything found in the car boot the worst scenario was they would not be seen outside their bathroom for a couple of days.

A discussion about animals and the ways they have involved me with criminals and the law would not be complete without referring briefly to animal cruelty. Like most vets in practice I have occasionally encountered cruelty so repulsive that I shall not attempt to describe it and thank the heavens that these encounters were very few and far between. As we all know, cruelty takes many forms and is sometimes the result of an owner killing their pet with kindness. The obese dog that is doomed to joint degeneration from an early age has been the subject of media attention for decades and still the obsessively kind owners continue to stuff their fat dogs with cream cakes, and perhaps they always will. At the other end of the spectrum is, of course, the malnutrition and starvation of animals as a result of the owner's stupidity.

All the cases in which I was involved over the years seemed to follow the same pattern. In the case of the greedy rogue farmer, he failed to provide adequate feed for the cattle or the sheep, and often combined his disregard with an appalling and unacceptable standard of husbandry. From time to time, it gave me great satisfaction to provide supporting evidence in court that led to their successful prosecution. With domestic pets the cruelty caused by neglect sometimes became apparent at the time it was necessary for some reason to examine the pets of initially well-intentioned people who simply had no funds to pay for a tin of cat or dog food. Often it was combined with not having enough money to provide for their numerous children. What do you say to such an owner, who asks, 'Why shouldn't my kids have animals just like everyone else?' There were times when I could have yelled at them, 'Because you can't bloomin' well afford them, that's why.' But I never did. The dilemma was that I knew that all the numerous children would in some way benefit from their family association with their pets, but sadly they could not with neglected animals like that.

Since I hung up my rugby boots, my Saturday afternoon violent aspirations have been limited to shouting in our Gloucester's Kingsholm stadium, usually at the referee. The point I am trying to make is that when senseless violence was inflicted on the animals I treated there was never a referee to help them. There was the odd owner who bullied their pet into submission in the belief that it was part of a strict training programme. Occasionally the act of cruelty was the result of an individual striking out or kicking an animal impulsively. This would often occur at night after the owner obviously had one too many. Enough said, you have heard it all before. Actually, you have not. There was one particular case woth relating.

The telephone rang late one Saturday night and a frightened lady asked me if I would look at their Labrador dog that had just been involved in a road accident. They believed he was concussed but was recovering. He needed to be seen anyway to ensure he had not received internal injuries, and within the half hour the Jones' arrived at the surgery with their dog, Joe. He was unsteady on his feet when I lifted him onto the table. I was surprised that I could not find a single superficial mark on him, but he was certainly not *compos mentis*. I remarked that this was odd and asked if they had actually seen the accident. The owners looked at one another, apparently knowing that I did not believe their story. Then the truth came out. Mr Jones' lips began to tremble and he had difficulty speaking. He put his arm around his wife's shoulders and sobbed.

'There wasn't an accident', he eventually managed to reveal, 'I hit him and I'm so sorry.'

Mr Jones certainly packed a punch. In the intervals when he was once more in control of himself he explained that they had been out for the evening and when they arrived home Joe had come to greet them and in his excitement jumped up against him. It must have been a bad night for Mr Jones. He responded by landing a severe uppercut on his dog, who was immediately knocked unconscious. Joe was steadily recovering on my examination table and I am sure the repeated apologies from a distressed Mr Jones to Joe cradled in his arms were reassuring enough to mend any bond, which must have been stretched to breaking point. But clearly a bond existed between them.

The young couple came to see me the next day, and of course tail-wagging Joe was with them. Apologies all round were still abundant. All was well and by now they were appreciated but unnecessary. I suspect that the owners may have been anxious to know if there were 'further enquiries' to be made in a case like this. Was this a case of cruelty? I am not a judge, but until today I have never told anyone about what actually happened that night. I was satisfied it would never happen again.

Another example of madness is the sort I really wish we would never see again, but I have not sufficient faith in human nature to believe that. These events happened a long time ago and the area in Churchdown where this took place has changed immensely for the better. One afternoon a middle-aged couple came into surgery with a small kitten who was fitting. Within minutes of a clinical examination it was clear that it had meningitis resulting from head trauma. The couple had witnessed a group of youths playing a ball game with the cat outside a block of flats. One young lad took the cat up the stairs to a higher balcony and tossed it to other members of the group waiting below. If the unfortunate creature had had any luck someone would have caught him before he hit the ground. The state of the kitten showed that he had hit it on more than one occasion. This really was a shocking example of juvenile cruelty and I discussed the case the following day with the local RSPCA inspector.

Before continuing I need to make it clear that I am a member of the RSPCA and have been for most of my life. I support most of the society's policies and have much respect for the achievements of the dedicated, hardworking, fund-raising members, particularly at local level, from one end of the country to the other. My comments are not a criticism of the society, just of one inspector at a particular time in history whose ineptitude made me so angry and frustrated I cannot forget him. It will now not come as too much of a surprise when I say that I was a bit disappointed by the inspector's response. I was also astonished. Assuming it was his job to investigate cases of alleged cruelty to animals, he was being handed a case on a plate. He was given the names of the individuals dropping the cat from the balcony, the names of the witnesses and a veterinary report of the cat's injuries prior to euthanasia. He was not the slightest bit interested and I was flabbergasted.

'Well, do you think you could go along and have a word with the individuals concerned?'

'A waste of time, my man', was the reply. 'That lot are so used to talking to people in uniform it would be water off a duck's back', or ridiculous words to the same effect. As far as I was concerned he should have hung up his uniform there and then, but no doubt he would have continued to his impending retirement and a back-slapping session where someone else swathed in medals spoke of his lifetime's dedication to animal welfare. Thank the Lord for the present generation of RSPCA inspectors.

Towards the end of surgery one cold January morning my receptionist Claire tapped on my consulting room door and apologised for interrupting me.

'I am sorry to bother you, Mr Smith, but I've just taken a call from a client in Hucclecote and I think you should deal with this one as soon as you can.'

'Oh dear, what's the problem?' I replied in a nonchalant way, still looking forward to the first cup of surgery coffee of the day.

'I am not sure what has happened', she continued, 'but a horse has suffered a dreadful head injury.' An injury resulting from a road traffic accident immediately came to mind, but Claire was sure that there were no vehicles involved.

'Okay, ring him back and reassure him I'll be with him in just a few minutes.'

The patient was a small sixteen-year-old Welsh Mountain pony called Bubbles. Her owners were Bryn and Janet Rudge who lived in Hucclecote and stabled the pony in a small building on the slopes of Chosen Hill. Local children enjoyed rides on her around the lower fields of the hill, and many others simply went to say hello. Who on earth could possibly wish her any harm?

I met an ashen-faced Bryn in the field near the little stable. He tried to prepare me for what I was about to see but his words were totally inadequate. Blood was splattered all around the small stable building, and a closer inspection revealed tiny fragments of skin and hair. In the centre of the carnage Bubbles stood motionless. She was unrecognisable as a pony. Her head had been beaten to a pulp. Her face was so flattened and distorted that her features were more like those of a donkey. I am sure no further description is necessary for anyone to appreciate the full horror of it. Words of comfort to her were a waste of time; she was dying.

I rang my old colleagues at Ormond Eeles and had a quick chat with Walter's son, Richard. I knew that he would not be long coming but if Bubbles was still aware of anything a few minutes would be a very long time. I gave her a massive dose of pethidine and she sank to the floor shortly afterwards. We waited. I looked around the building and did not have to look far to find the murder weapon – on the floor at one end was a sticky, bloodstained scaffold pole. Richard walked into the stable and uttered, 'Good God, I hadn't expected this.' Neither of us had. Surely nothing other than a battlefield could create such a scene. Richard raised his gun to Bubbles' head. There was a sharp bang and she suffered no more. Sadly I had watched Richard, or his sister's husband, Bob, perform this humane killing on many occasions. It was remarkably professional. It was fast, safe and accurate and the stress on both horse and owner was kept to a minimum. At the appropriate moment the gun seemed to deftly appear from nowhere and in the next second it was all over.

The following day back at my surgery our local RSPCA inspector, Alan Brockbank, called in for a chat about the incident. He too joined the ranks of those who had never seen or heard the likes of it. A reward for information was offered at the time but as far as I am aware no one was ever arrested for the crime. That was seventeen years ago. It's hard to believe that the person who carried out this atrocity has lived with this on their conscience all this time.

On a happier note and once more side-tracking from the animals, it is a pleasure to write about the Rudge family of Hucclecote. Peter and Edward (Teddy) Rudge were classmates from the time we donned our maroon Crypt School blazers in 1952. Peter and I often asked each other, 'Where did Ted get his brains from?' He had IQ to spare. We were fortunate enough to have a maths master in school at the time named Arthur C. 'Aggie' Paget. He was reputed to be the best mathematician ever to be associated with the Crypt School. That was of course before Teddy came along. Which one was the more brilliant? I cannot answer that one. I don't think I was suitably placed to judge, except on those occasions when I found myself at a desk near him in an end of term exam.

At some stage I was taught additional maths, which embraced calculus, and it was not long before I thought I was being taught another language. I was never close enough to read what Ted had written, just near enough to see how much he had written. While I struggled to get beyond my fifth line of deductions I could see he had filled one side of foolscap, and I was convinced we could not have been given the same question. Ted was never destined to be a schoolteacher but how I benefited from his knowledge of A-level physics and chemistry. His enthusiasm for these subjects made him a natural teacher and he appeared to have more patience than our officially appointed ones.

When it came to the crunch we did not do too badly in our final school exams. I was not awarded the school's prestigious Townsend Scholarship or a State Scholarship in Mathematics and Physics which was tenable at Queen's College Cambridge. That accolade went to Edward Rudge.

I had my place at the Liverpool Vet School and that was what I wanted.

CHAPTER TWELVE

CLOSING REFLECTIONS

All stories have to end at some point. I began to write mine during the cold wintry days of 2007. For several years now I have enjoyed being part of Churchdown's Local History Society. At school I had no interest in the darned subject but as i grew older I became obsessed with it. You could call it an age thing I suppose. Anne Boden, the society's 'never take a break' chairman, thought that I could give an interesting talk that revolved around my veterinary career in the village that now spanned decades. Anne and her family had been clients almost from the time I put up my plate in 1972. I gave the talk, and by chance that night a young commissioning editor from a local publishing company was in the audience. She believed I had some experiences others might be interested to read about and asked if I had considered writing a book of veterinary memoirs. So I did, and if you have managed to get this far I hope you have enjoyed my memories of life in the Cotswolds and its animal (and human) inhabitants.

Writing the book was trickier than the talk. Which of the hundreds of rewarding, disappointing, happy, sad or simply ridiculous memories are of interest to readers? There is so much to tell and no chairman to tell you when to stop talking. The veterinary memories are not just of my patients; most of the unforgettable stories arose from a situation created by the innocent actions of an owner and their interactions with their pet. My last chapter ends with just a few memorable cases from my career.

At the start of my career, my Vet School demanded that I spend a number of weeks working each vacation, always for free, at stables and farms to gain experience in horse and farm husbandry and management. This offered me a unique opportunity to spend time at the stables at our local pub, the Wagon & Horses, and I was in some ways privileged to be accepted there. At the same time the stable owners were happy for me to be there, mucking out for nothing. On the bright side it was part of my education and it kept me fit, and those few weeks were a real education. I toiled hard when the bosses were around and chatted to the locals and stable girls when they were not. It was also convenient for me to see horse practice there during the day and to see Angela at night. Her family home was just down the road and she was by now my fiancée: engaged to be married to a penniless student.

The stables had been managed for a very long time by Mr Llewellyn-Jones and his business partner Gerald Brown. Both men were horse experts in different ways. Mr Brown was keen to teach me horse and stable management and I learnt a great deal from him. I learnt a lot too from Mr Llewellyn-Jones. It is not so easy to describe his equine speciality, perhaps 'a study of the things that they will not teach you at Vet School' might be close to the mark. Before I had been formally instructed at Liverpool to age horses by their teeth, Mr Llewellyn-Jones had already taught me the ways in which the apparent age of the horse could be altered with a dental rasp and a bit of chicanery. By the time I had been taught the significance of a 'seven-year-hook' on an upper corner incisor of a seven-year-old horse, I knew how to remove it.

Two of the most important health aspects of buying and selling horses are ensuring that the horse is sound in wind and limb. A lame horse that cannot breathe properly is of little use to anyone. The old sage nevertheless was aware of methods of minimising nasal discharges and the low-grade chronic lameness that temporarily disappeared with a gentle warming-up exercise prior to a sale inspection. I am sure that he never indulged in this sort of cunning himself of course, and it was thoughtful of him to pass some of his wealth of knowledge on to me. As a young professional, I found the examination of a horse for soundness on behalf of a purchaser to be one of the most onerous of routine jobs. I often lay in bed at night wondering what imperceptible sign of some impending problem the horse might have had that I had missed that day.

An occasion I remember well was the evening John Harvey rang. John is still a large local sheep farmer at Walton Cardiff, near Tewkesbury, now vastly developed. Like most of us, his rugby-playing days are now just memories. I would bet that one of his adrenalin rushes was the evening he scored a winning try playing for Cheltenham's Old Pats in a 1960s Rugby Cup Final. It was a gigantic effort from the biggest, if not the fastest, forward on the field. On this occasion John wanted *me* to move fast. There had been a freak accident when his daughter's pony had jumped a fence and a fractured pole had speared his posterior abdomen. The jagged point had entered the inguinal region, traversed the body and emerged through the gluteal muscles of the hindquarter.

Somehow, miraculously, the pole had missed the numerous major nerves and blood vessels in the region, and the internal organs, and if it had struck the bony pelvis it had been deflected from it. At the time I drew up the Immobilon I was not sure of any of this. I sawed through the pole to shorten it, cleaned and disinfected it as thoroughly as possible and eased it gradually out of the anaesthetised horse's body.

Back in the farmhouse kitchen, over a cup of coffee, we discussed the possible complications that might arise over the next few days. The pony came round rapidly from the anaesthetic and was recovering well from the ordeal. With the help of a great concentration of antibiotics and other appropriate injections, the wounds healed well and remarkably he was soon back in action as though this alarming episode had never happened.

Regrettably not all emergencies have happy endings and one I have never been able to forget began one Monday morning on my way to our Brockworth surgery. When I reached the Ermin Street junction a tanker lorry was stationary at an odd angle in the road, and it was surrounded by a crowd of anxious-looking people. I arrived at the same time as a police car and, after a brief discussion, said I was happy to crawl under the lorry to attend to a Collie dog that was unable to scramble from under the lorry. He was unable to stand and in his frightened state did not at all appreciate me wanting to move him. I slipped a muzzle over his jaws and eased him on to a blanket. We slowly dragged the blanket away from the underside of the lorry and transferred him to my car, and within minutes he was lying on my surgery table. It was important to assess the extent of his injuries as quickly as possible and when I left the surgery at Brockworth I took my heavily sedated patient with me.

Back at Churchdown I anaesthetised him and X-rayed his back, his pelvis and his hind limbs to find the reason he could not stand. It was fairly obvious. His pelvis was fractured, a femur was fractured and the tibia in the same leg was in no better shape. His injuries were dreadful but nevertheless, given enough time, they were probably all treatable and with the aid of pins, plates and screws, the injuries could be repaired. We were now at the stage where we would be able to explain the situation to his anxious owner, what needed to be done to put things right, and not unimportantly, what it was going to cost. I felt sure that by the end of the day the worried owner of this plucky dog would be there to claim him. Then the client would have to be told that the final fees would, at today's value, be around £1,000. You hoped they would respond with 'Thank Heaven he's insured.'

Therein lay a problem. It was not that he was uninsured, but a couple of days later we had not found an owner, despite the many announcements and coverage on local radio and the newspapers. Nobody seemed to want him. I suspect that a nurse had detected a growing bond between me and this dog, and she suggested, 'Why don't you have him, Mr Smith?' The persuasion continued: 'He would make a lovely pal for Jimmy.' The thought had crossed my mind.

There would be a great deal of surgical work involved and it would be expensive to the practice in materials and time but it would be my time, and time was now of the essence. There was an optimum interval for commencing orthopaedic work following the injuries and we had already passed that while we waited for the owners to come and claim their dog. Friday came and went. Under different circumstances I would have been delighted. It was not my on-duty weekend and on Monday, yippee, we were off on our family holiday. It was a huge dilemma, and I realised that, not for the first time, I had become the judge and the jury.

I weighed up all the factors. I would have to delegate the surgical work, and there was an awful lot of it, to the assistant vet or even the locum who may have relished the challenge or may have resented the apparent obligation. There were endless possibilities of complications that could arise and, rightly or wrongly, I began to realise that my heart was ruling my head and I decided to put the dog to sleep.

I went into surgery on the Sunday night, looked into his eyes with more than a little feeling of failure, and painlessly injected the barbiturate. I was glad on this occasion that for some reason the nurses had not given this affectionate stray a name. We never did have a chance to find out what name someone else had given him.

Defining what is an emergency is not always an easy task. Even in today's enlightened world the telephone will ring in the middle of the night and at the other end is the owner of a young female cat, suddenly rolling in apparent agony with acute abdominal pain. There is a 99 per cent chance that telling the distraught owner that 'what she needs is the attention of a tomcat to put her right' is not the sort of reply they are expecting to hear from the vet at 3 a.m. So I often found myself carrying out a full clinical examination of the super-affectionate cat which had suddenly come into season just in case I was 1 per cent wrong.

But what is an emergency call? From my own experience here is one snippet of advice for the new graduate vet. If the owner believes it is an emergency, it is an emergency, and they were not always wrong. I recall a time when a simple bitch spay could have turned into an emergency had not one of the owners insisted that the daft young Churchdown vet must have given stupid advice. The Friday morning operation had been quite routine. There had been no complications and in normal fashion the patient was discharged at the end of the day with the usual instructions, which included 'no solids by mouth for 24 hours', plus, 'Come back on Monday for a check-up and in ten days for the stitches to be removed.'

It was about the fourth day when the wife rang up to query the post-operative instructions. 'Surely this cannot be right?' she questioned the receptionist. 'My dog hasn't had any food this week, she's ravenous and she cannot possibly just survive on fluids for the next ten days.' There had quite clearly been a misunderstanding. After four days without food their dog was starving. This certainly was not the message I had intended to convey to her German husband. His English was poor and my German was non-existent. I could cope with a little French and understood Forest of Dean. All's well that ends well and at the end of the ten days the chubby little Dachshund happily rolled over to show off her hysterectomy wound for the removal of her stitches.

I will never forget Paddy either, a sprightly Irish Setter who couldn't go too long without an obligatory trip to the vet, and his track record suggested that it was just a matter of time before he was involved in an emergency of one kind or another. It happened about lunchtime on a beautiful hot summer's day. Paddy's owner was an experienced nurse at a local hospital and earlier that morning she retired to rest after a night on duty. While she put her head down Paddy stretched out in the garden and did likewise. Now most dogs would by nature choose a cool shady spot to sleep. He must have selected a south-facing wall, and when he woke, he was hot, very hot. Nurse Avril rang at 1 p.m. She knew he was in trouble this time, and he was already showing the very serious early signs of heatstroke. Full blown heatstroke was not an uncommon problem in surgery when we saw some warm weather.

A typical scenario was the collapsed, exhausted pet brought into surgery panting madly and becoming increasingly comatose. The diagnosis was usually self-evident, and often followed a marathon over Chosen Hill on a tropical summer afternoon. It was sometimes difficult to explain to a devoted incredulous owner that no matter what we did now he may still not recover. Hospitalisation and intensive care, intravenous fluids by the litre, heart drugs and steroids to help prevent brain damage might be essential, but at the top of the list of immediate needs was a cold water bath.

Before I left the surgery for her house, I asked Avril to start running a cold bath, and ten minutes later we carried a confused, floppy, gasping Paddy upstairs to the bathroom. When I had taken his temperature the mercury seemed to be trying to escape, but we would soon lower it. With one last heave we shoved him into the cold water and immersed him so that just his head was a little above the surface. We knew he was beginning to recover when he decided to get out, so we shoved him back in again. After several rounds of getting in and out, and on each occasion it became a bigger effort to keep him in, we assumed he was getting better, and by now we were both almost as wet as the patient. He made a complete recovery.

I suppose most wives would question their husband's behaviour if they arrived home from work dripping wet. Angela was used to me appearing at any time of the day dishevelled and in some sort of disarray, and took it for granted. Just another day at the office.

The stories roll on and, regrettably, so do the years. The Brambles surgery that we had created in the 1970s had steadily grown and the original surgery building had reached the size of a large bungalow but even so, by the end of the '90s, it was simply too small to accommodate the ever-increasing staff and to provide the facilities that we needed to maintain the standard of service to a greater number of our clients that I had always strived for. I was lucky enough to secure the derelict old cottages on the opposite side of the road and with the aid of both a very good architect and a local builder transformed a blot on the landscape into a state-of-the-art surgery.

Angela and I were appreciative and perhaps even took a little pride in what we had achieved in those thirty years, but we were not getting any younger and we began to ask ourselves – what next? Perhaps we were subconsciously looking for a new challenge. At some stage others would have to take over the practice, and thoughts, followed by talk of retirement began to surface. The millennium was approaching and it came and went without anything much happening other than fireworks at midnight. The decision however was made, and now already (unbelievably) sixty, I retired in the spring of 2001. It coincided with the worst that nature had to offer: the biggest outbreak of Foot and Mouth Disease the country has known.

I am sure the dreadful events of that time are still fixed in the minds of many people as clearly as in mine. The slaughter and the sight of the bodies of the dead cattle and sheep piled high in the fields, the stench of the pyres and the distress it caused to the farming community will never leave one's mind. Inevitably at times the stress of it all brought out the worst in people, and sometimes farmers behaved in unpredictable ways. My scariest moment occurred near Blakeney Hill in the Forest of Dean. One day I stopped my car in response to a thickset local chap who appeared to be waving me down, no doubt to give me helpful directions to a little farm that I could not find. This Forester seemed to know instinctively who I was and where I had come from. He walked slowly to the nearside of my car and an angry red face appeared through the window I had fully opened, perhaps unwisely. His initial remarks were not too welcoming, and he made his point quickly.

'You're a friggin' vet, aren't you?' It was more of a statement than a question.

'You're from friggin' MAFF.' I cannot remember whether I actually got round to saying anything at all to him, but his inquisition and his venomous lecture to me on what we were all doing wrong continued, and his big fist was uncomfortably close to my neck.

In his defence I suspect this temporarily demented chap who had given me a vicious tongue-lashing was acting out of character. Later I discovered he had already had his sheep destroyed and meeting me gave him the opportunity to take his feelings out on a Ministry official. Eventually he stood back and I was able to raise the window, probably after I had nodded an assurance that I would forward his recommendations to the Divisional Veterinary Officers at Elmbridge Court. He seemed to know them all by name.

I was a TVI, a Temporary Veterinary Inspector, and there were scores of us up and down the country. At the start of the outbreak MAFF was hopelessly undermanned and to fill the gap quickly an army of retired vets were asked to volunteer for service, and the Last of the Summer Wine responded. As so often in these situations, much of our work was of a very routine nature, and was combined not unexpectedly with the traditional government paperwork in triplicate. Nevertheless, most of us found it surprisingly interesting, and I think we did a reasonable job. Most importantly we took the pressure off the permanent MAFF staff and possibly our humour kept their spirits up.

Within weeks of the start of the outbreak many of the senior MAFF people were looking drained and some did become quite ill under the strain. We took our work seriously, but as you can imagine in circumstances like these, there were often opportunities to swap tales with other TVIs and to enjoy the company of colleagues that you had not seen for years. All had experiences to relate, many were horrible but some were amusing. I was very pleasantly surprised to meet a vet there who was an old boy from my school, a very well-known one in fact. He was Old Cryptian Bryan 'Grunter' Green.

After he qualified Bryan had worked in a large Gloucester farm practice and as a schoolboy I had 'seen practice' with him. In his younger days he had been much more than your average local rugby player and I had enjoyed watching him turn out for Gloucester at Kingsholm when I was still a youngster at the Crypt School. Murphy's law had prevented him getting an England cap. He had been selected to play in the final England trial but a cow kicked him at an inappropriate time; he fractured a collarbone and missed the game. Bryan had travelled from Sussex to join the Dad's Army of TVIs where he had practised for most of his working life. He is a big chap but he met his match in the Forest of Dean on one occasion.

A small lady resisted his attempts to enter her farm and the confrontation that followed ended with her chucking a bucket of disinfectant over him. Retaliation was out of the question. This wet episode was not Swansea or Ebbw Vale on a wintry Saturday afternoon. He knew how to deal with assaults down there. That was where you got your retaliation in first, of course.

Having led an active life I wondered, as I am sure everyone does, how I would adapt to life in retirement. Enjoying the beautiful Gloucestershire countryside without one ear listening out for the telephone was a new experience. Simply wandering around the village was a fresh pleasure, and Sunday mornings could be particularly rewarding and entertaining. It was remarkable to see what the youngsters could do on a steep ramp whilst balanced on a narrow skateboard. Now, simply walking with Coco around the nearby playing fields became very much a social occasion. It was wonderful to have time just to chat with the pet owners I had only talked to across an examination table for years. The vast majority of the owners are responsible folk who take clearing up their dogs' droppings seriously but there are the arrogant ones who still believe the rules do not apply to them and their dogs. They drove me wild.

For many fellows, Sunday morning was the time for the weekly game of football, and the players too added something of interest to the Sunday morning walk in the village, and for sheer entertainment value some of the games were second to none. It was not exactly David Beckham standard but the enthusiasm was top class. One morning a football whizzed past the goalpost and landed near where I was watching the match with my dog. While the goalie was having a heated argument with his full-back, Coco nose-dribbled the ball back on to the field of play.

The goalie shouted to the full-back to get off the pitch and let the dog take his place as it was a better player than he was. We discreetly moved quickly out of harm's way and minutes later were at the other end of the field. On this occasion the ball shot cleanly between the other goalie's legs and his side went hysterical. The goal scorer did not seem to object to the embraces he was getting from some of his forwards and then, after what seemed a ritual 'give me five' sort of handshake with everybody, he decided to do a celebratory acrobatic turn. It bore little resemblance to the Premiership double back-flip and land on your feet sort of thing. Nevertheless I was impressed as he took off and did a spectacular diving bellyflop into the mud. While he was in mid-air I prayed he would not land in anything else.

For the first two or three years it was wonderful to be able to wander over Chosen Hill and enjoy the many other lovely walks in the Cotswolds, naturally at that time always accompanied by Coco. Our daughter, Sally, had moved to Derbyshire so the opportunity to walk in the Peak District as well arose. With the added pleasure of the company of her new chocolate Labrador pal Bramble, we roamed for endless miles. But nothing lasts for ever and eventually the ever-youthful Coco began to show signs of her age catching up with her.

One weekend Angela was spending a few days with Sally when there was a sudden and unexpected deterioration in Coco's health. Her kidney function had gradually started to fail but for the last year I had managed to control it well and she enjoyed a happy and active life. Things were clearly not right on the Saturday morning. She was strangely subdued and was content to sleep for most of the day, only venturing into the garden when I went out for a stroll. Stopping for a quick drink at the pond was normal behaviour for her, but on this occasion she stopped and lapped and gave the impression she did not really know what she wanted to do. I took a small blood sample from her and ran through the same kidney function tests that I had regularly monitored. I was astounded by the deterioration. Poor Coco was developing the acute phase of renal failure. It was time for intensive care and a great deal of fluid therapy and medication to reverse what was happening, and with this immense effort, stress and confusion to her there was a strong likelihood that there would be more of the same for her within days. In my heart I knew we were approaching the end of the road.

I was up early Sunday morning. The morning sun after the overnight frosts in February are too good to miss, but I suppose the real reason was to check on the dear old dog. She looked up as I opened the door of the utility and her weak tail attempted a wag. She struggled to follow me as I walked slowly up the garden. Already she seemed to be in another world. I carried her back into the house where she slept for a few hours. The routine was repeated in the afternoon but this time, when I turned to walk back to the house, she did not follow me. I left her on the lawn and watched her behaviour with interest. Her head rose and she sniffed the air. She appeared contented and slowly began to make her way back. Bravely she carefully descended a few stone steps that led to the garden pond. She stopped and attempted to reach forward to drink. Her forelimbs were too weak to support her and she stumbled and struggled to avoid falling into the water. She was losing her dignity, albeit in the secluded garden that she loved. I was choked and could watch no more, and I carried her into the house for the last time.

It was the middle of the afternoon and I had made the decision. I telephoned Angela and in a shaky voice broke the news to her. She asked if I wanted her to return straight away but, the decision made, I wanted to do the necessary as quickly as possible. Still in some way I wanted Angela to be there at the end of Coco's life. She listened sadly to my intentions which she knew I would carry out. At 5 o'clock Angela was aware that I was giving our dog a heavy sedative injection, and probably she could envisage me lifting her on to the kitchen counter an hour later and giving the final injection. Coco died at 6 o'clock. At first light the next morning I dug her grave in the hard white ground and laid her to rest. Later, I packed a case and drove north to Derbyshire, alone. On arrival it was sad to see Bramble charging around, jumping in and out of our car excitedly searching for his mate, and it was many months before that behaviour pattern was broken.

We made the move to Derbyshire in the summer of 2007 and now enjoy a quiet relaxing life in beautiful countryside. Well, it is quiet until the granddaughters arrive. But when Angela is engaged with them, nothing gives me greater pleasure than to walk with Bramble in this peaceful area of lanes, fields, peaks and rivers. At these times I often think of all that has happened over the years and the people I still vividly recall.

Tragically, out of the blue, our close friend John Eggleton suffered a fatal heart attack and died in the summer of 2000. We had looked forward to numerous happy days in retirement together. Many of them would have been spent on the banks of rivers, most of the day perhaps just reminiscing or putting the world to rights, and if we caught fish that would be the usual bonus. The loss of John was shared, among innumerable friends, with another former classmate, Mike Greening. The three of us had fished together as schoolboys and enjoyed each other's company for almost half a century. At the end of his professional career with the Civil Service, Mike retired and we meet up regularly at Kingsholm. We are still able to spend the occasional day together angling, and you can be certain that at some time during the fishing day one of us will ask, 'Do you remember that day we went with John to —?' Neither of us will forget that day, no matter which one it was.

Julian Pettifer, the son of the principal of my first practice in Crudwell, is still a very active globe-trotting broadcaster cum writer/journalist. His reports from Vietnam won him the BAFTA Reporter of the Year Award in 1968. Today he occasionally hosts Gardener's Question Time on Radio 4, a far more sensible occupation than dodging bullets in Vietnam. He is still infuriatingly good looking.

What happened to Hubert Evans of Crudwell fame? Believe it or not he did die with his boots on, just as Angela's mother had predicted. However I am sure she did not envisage it happening behind a cow. Poor Taff turned out one night to attend the animal in Ashton Keynes that was having difficulty calving. I can imagine the scenario, and if ever there was a worse place to encounter an obstetrical problem for Hubert this must have been it, in the company of one his most demanding clients. We last had the opportunity to meet up with Taff at a disco held at Cirencester's Rugby Club. It was several years after we had left his Crudwell practice and we had bumped into each other at a Cotswold Veterinary Surgeons' Society meeting in Cheltenham. He was very amiable, and being his usual persuasive self, insisted that we should go along. Taff was at his social best at the dance and proudly introduced us to his vet assistants.

'I don't suppose you knew I had two assistants now, did you?' He tried very hard to mention this monumental fact in the most casual way possible. Angela's response was spontaneous and totally out of character. She replied, 'So you don't do any work at all now then, Mr Evans?' He for once was lost for words.

I was immensely fortunate as a new graduate to have been associated with John Bourne in my first job. I saw a great deal of him in my first year and learned a huge amount from him. He set the benchmark standard, and knowing what was expected of me I quickly gained the confidence to be a good farm animal vet and packed a lot of experience into a short space of time. John had left the practice in Crudwell to take up a teaching and research post at the School of Veterinary Science at Bristol University. He rapidly rose through the academic ranks and in recent years Professor F.J. Bourne has been chairman of the Independent Scientific Group, the ISG, on cattle TB. I am only able to mention in passing the opposing views on how we should be controlling the spread of bovine TB. Everyone is in agreement that the badger is involved in the spread of the disease. The argument in its simplistic form is, what do you do about it?

The majority of practising vets and most farmers are convinced that culling the badgers is essential to bring bovine TB under control. The ISG concluded that badger culling can make no meaningful contribution to the control of cattle TB in Britain. And now our government's chief scientific adviser, and £40 million later, has chosen to ignore the years of research and the advice of the ISG, and has recommended a badger cull anyway. Are you confused?

I enjoyed the company of Mark Hicks-Beach both professionally on the farm and as a true friend, but life can be cruel and often inexplicable. Mark was fifty-five when he died in 1998. His death followed a short but very serious illness and today he still watches over the wonderful historic estate from the ancient cemetery at Witcombe Church.

Steve Butterworth, the young assistant who joined The Brambles practice in 1988, brought a new dimension of veterinary orthopaedics to the area. A top job opportunity unexpectedly arose in the orthopaedic department at the Bristol Vet School and Steve sadly left Churchdown to take up the prestigious post at the university. He left behind high practice standards, many photographs of his interesting work, and pictures of his upturned car in a Brockworth field. Today he is the principal of one of the UK's specialist vet orthopaedic referral practices in Swansea.

There have been so many farmers and pet owners and some 'I'm not sure actually where you fit in' type characters that I could write about. I hope I have represented everyone fairly. No? Well, I have done my best and don't expect everyone to agree.

Most of my Liverpool Vet School year of 1960 have now of course retired. I regret that it has not been possible to write about each one of them. You would never believe some of the stories anyway. At some time in my life they have all played an important role and I am very lucky to have enjoyed their company in a very special way. Graham, our wonderfully talented and tolerant Stroud chauffeur, has enjoyed a brilliant career working for the government's Veterinary Services, and at last he has been persuaded to retire. My old flatmates Nigel and Roger have spent most of their professional lives as practice principals in Lancashire practices and are now enjoying a quieter pace of life, some of the time. Between them, they enjoy walking, painting, reading newspapers, wine tasting, beer tasting, golf, watching afternoon television and eating out. They also still enjoy playing the guitar! Who in their right mind would want to be friends with sixty-plus-year-old rockers buying Gibson and Fender guitars? Actually it's still great fun and occasionally I'm invited to one of their jam sessions. Never thought 'When I'm Sixty-Four' would come around so soon. Nigel has recently formed a Rotarians' Rock Group. Wait for it – they are the 'Elderly Brothers'.

Wynn Walters has hung his wellies up at last. He left the Cheltenham practice in 1971 and since then many Wiltshire and Cotswold farmers have enjoyed his company and professionalism. He remains one of our pals at vet gatherings who are still there late in the evening long after the others have retired to bed, happy to reminisce around a log fire. Bonded to most of the youngsters who met by chance at a vet school in 1960 these old friends start to become inseparable from the relatives. Compared to the much larger numbers of students who enter vet school today, we were indeed a very small band starting together, just twenty-nine chaps and six young ladies. How times have changed. The proportion of women entering vet schools today can be in excess of 80 per cent.

Already we have sadly lost several of the men from natural causes. For different reasons two of the losses I have special reason to mention. A popular chap in our year was Fred Tomusange. He hailed from Uganda and, at thirty-two, was the oldest in the year when we began our course. We enjoyed his company and that of his wife and young children for the five years we spent together in Liverpool. On qualifying he returned to Uganda and we know that he was soon an important member of the Ugandan government's Agriculture Department, the equivalent of the UK's DEFRA. Within a few years we lost all contact with Fred and our attempts to track him down were met with unhelpful replies from the Amin administration. None of us are sure but we feel that he may well have been one of the 500,000 Ugandans who mysteriously disappeared when President Idi Amin was in power.

Considering the academic pressures we were under and living closely in each others' company for most of the time I think we all got on superbly well together. Naturally for some reason or other we were all down in the dumps at times but together we kept our spirits high. A pint, a chat and a good laugh in the local Brook House pub on Smithdown Road, Liverpool, put everything into its true perspective. We maintained our youthful dignity and sanity, and we survived the course supporting each other. It was not until recent years that we thought perhaps we could have done more to have stopped one of our year from taking his own life. Suicide in our student and young postgraduate days was something so unlikely that nobody – as far as I know – would ever have given it a second thought. There was so much to live for. So how in Heaven's name can you now account for the veterinary profession being the top of the professional suicide league? The statistics are frightening.

Numerous suggestions and even scientific papers have been written to explain how this situation has arisen. I suspect we all have our own differing opinions on the reasons for this tragic state of affairs. Regardless, I find it sad that if recent surveys can be believed over half the vets in the profession wish that they had chosen a different career. Where has it all gone so terribly wrong?

I am pleased I became a vet and have few regrets, and even in retirement I still feel I am one. Today I enjoy the sound of the *Veterinary Record* dropping through the letterbox and thumbing the pages at the breakfast table, even if the job adverts are of no interest. I have enjoyed my career and I have had the good fortune to meet hundreds of wonderful people and their animals. Some of the clients, in one way or other, produced more than their share of good humour and laughter. One such chap was Peter Stubbs, whose family had run the 'open all hours' store on Cheltenham Road East in Churchdown.

Gloucester has been fortunate to retain its four ancient grammar schools despite decades of political pressure to abolish them. The affectionate rivalry between the two boys' schools is memorable and regularly results in friendly banter at social gatherings. Peter was not an Old Cryptian. He went to the other school, Sir Thomas Rich's, and he reminded me of it on every occasion I called to fill up with petrol. At the shop you could buy a loaf of bread, a tin of polish and probably the 'fork 'andles' or 'four candles' as well. However, a ten-minute chat with proprietor Peter was obligatory when we put the world of Gloucester rugby and what was wrong in the village to rights, usually in that order. One afternoon a mutual customer who owned a big Rottweiler cross called into the shop and tied his dog to the handle of a large dustbin. While the customary debate was in progress, the Rotty spied his rival, Rover, on the other side of the main road. Not to be hampered by being tied to a big bin he took off, dragging the noisy missile behind him. Screeching brakes broke up the argument on who should play in the front row.

It was unfortunate that this should happen at the time of day when traffic was pouring out of the Dowty Rotol factory, and it was just as busy on the Gloucester side of the traffic lights at the Hare & Hounds pub. The sight of the dustbin whizzing along behind a big dog determined to say hello to Rover on the opposite side must have been astonishing. The bewildered owner was confronted with trying to sort out a situation that resembled a scene from *Keystone Kops*. Whenever he shouted 'Come' another collision occurred a few seconds later. There was no serious harm to either of the animals involved and no doubt the dents, scratches and scrapes inflicted on the numerous vehicles that were skidding and swerving and bumping into each other were soon put right.

Moving to Churchdown was a defining moment in our lives and having lived there for so long we have wonderful memories. Unbelievably, and unbeknownst to me, so had my ancestors. One of the most fascinating time-consuming hobbies you can enjoy in retirement is researching your family history. I was surprised to find that my great-grandmother was an immediate descendant of Churchdown's Gaze family, and even more surprised to discover that my sixth great-grandfather, Emanuel, is buried at St Bartholomew's churchyard on Chosen Hill. He has actually got one of the best seats in the house, a short distance from the church's front door.

When I first visited his grave, I was astonished to find an inscription informing us that his eldest son, William, was 'killed by natives, Swan River Island, June 17th, 1832'. I was delighted to find that my great-uncle had gone to Western Australia as a 'Pioneer Settler' and not as a convict. His story is extremely well documented. William and a colleague were farming on the banks of the River Canning one day when they were attacked by a party of raiding Aborigines, led by a man named Yagan. William was speared five times but was still alive when he was rescued. He died from his wounds five days later, and during that time he made his will, the first to be proved in the Court of Western Australia. A bounty was put on Yagan's head, and he was hunted down and shot two years later. He then truly lost his head, which was smoked to preserve it before being transported to England. Amazingly it was housed in the Liverpool Museum and I must have walked past it most days when I attended Liverpool University in the '60s. Following a huge petition from the Aborigines, his head was returned in 1997 and today a large statue immortalising Yagan the freedom fighter stands on Swan River Island. And now you know why Chapter Five is entitled 'Pioneer Settlers'.

William's sixth great-nephew and his wife left for Derbyshire in August 2007, and Angela and I settled into our new rural home. At breakfast time, which these days is a very casual affair, we enjoy watching the mad behaviour of the large brown hares across the nearby fields, and we are visited by partridges and pheasants each morning. In the afternoons we are regularly visited by granddaughters Darcey and Millie. These tend to be far less tranquil occasions.

The Derbyshire countryside is beautiful, challenging and peaceful and we are fortunate to have lived in two beautiful parts of rural England. We enjoy our frequent trips to visit relatives and old friends in the Cotswolds. Invariably the conversation turns to the world of animals, and I am often asked, 'If you had the chance to do the same thing all over again, would you do it?'

There is only one answer:

You bet your life I would!